BLACKWELL

UNDERGROUND CLINICAL VIGNETTES

INTERNAL MEDICINE II: DERMATOLOGY, ID, NEPHROLOGY, UROLOGY, PULMONARY, RHEUMATOLOGY

BLACKWELL

UNDERGROUND CLINICAL VIGNETTES

INTERNAL MEDICINE II: DERMATOLOGY, ID, NEPHROLOGY, UROLOGY, PULMONARY, RHEUMATOLOGY

VIKAS BHUSHAN, MD
Series Editor
University of California, San Francisco, Class of 1991
Diagnostic Radiologist

VISHAL PALL, MD, MPH
Series Editor
Internist and Preventive Medicine Specialist
Government Medical College, Chandigarh – Panjab University – India, Class of 1997
Graduate School of Biomedical Sciences at UTMB Galveston, MPH, Class of 2004

TAO LE, MD
University of California, San Francisco, Class of 1996

ALIREZA KHAZAEIZADEH, MD
Shiraz University School of Medicine, Class of 1995
Associate Professor, Department of Biochemistry,
St. Luke's University School of Medicine

BAHAR SEDARATI, MD
Shiraz University School of Medicine, Class of 1995
Associate Professor, Department of Pathology,
St. Luke's University School of Medicine

Blackwell
Publishing

© 2005 by Blackwell Publishing

Blackwell Publishing, Inc., 350 Main Street, Malden, Massachusetts 02148-5018, USA
Blackwell Publishing Ltd, 9600 Garsington Road, Oxford OX4 2DQ, UK
Blackwell Publishing Asia Pty Ltd, 550 Swanston Street, Carlton, Victoria 3053, Australia

05 06 07 08 5 4 3 2 1

ISBN-13: 978-1-4051-0421-0
ISBN-10: 1-4051-0421-X

Library of Congress Cataloging-in-Publication Data

Internal medicine / Vikas Bhushan . . . [et al.]. — 3rd ed.
   v. ; cm. — (Blackwell underground clinical vignettes)
   "USMLE step 2 review."
   Contents: 1. Cardiology, endocrinology, GI, hem/onc — 2. Dermatology, ID, nephrology, urology, pulmonary, rheumatology.
   ISBN-13: 978-1-4051-0420-3 (pbk. : v. 1 : alk. paper)
   ISBN-10: 1-4051-0420-1 (pbk. : v. 1 : alk. paper)
   ISBN-13: 978-1-4051-0421-0 (pbk. : v. 2 : alk. paper)
   ISBN-10: 1-4051-0421-X (pbk. : v. 2 : alk. paper)
   1. Internal medicine—Case studies. 2. Physicians—Licenses—United States—Examinations—Study guides. I. Bhushan, Vikas. II. Series: Blackwell's underground clinical vignettes.
   [DNLM: 1. Internal Medicine—Case Reports. 2. Internal Medicine—Problems and Exercises. WB 18.2 I6122 2005]
   RC66.I576 2005
   616'.0076—dc22

2005009484

A catalogue record for this title is available from the British Library

Acquisitions: Nancy Anastasi Duffy
Development and Production: Debra Murphy
Cover and Interior Design: Leslie Haimes
Typesetter: Graphicraft in Quarry Bay, Hong Kong
Printed and bound by Capital City Press in Berlin, VT

For further information on Blackwell Publishing, visit our website:
www.blackwellmedstudent.com

NOTICE

The indications and dosages of all drugs in this book have been recommended in the medical literature and conform to the practices of the general community. The medications described do not necessarily have specific approval by the Food and Drug Administration for use in the diseases and dosages for which they are recommended. The package insert for each drug should be consulted for use and dosage as approved by the FDA. Because standards for usage change, it is advisable to keep abreast of revised recommendations, particularly those concerning new drugs.

The authors of this volume have taken care that the information contained herein is accurate and compatible with the standards generally accepted at the time of publication. Nevertheless, it is difficult to ensure that all the information given is entirely accurate for all circumstances. The publisher and authors do not guarantee the contents of this book and disclaim any liability, loss, or damage incurred as a consequence, directly or indirectly, of the use and application of any of the contents of this volume.

The publisher's policy is to use permanent paper from mills that operate a sustainable forestry policy, and which has been manufactured from pulp processed using acid-free and elementary chlorine-free practices. Furthermore, the publisher ensures that the text paper and cover board used have met acceptable environmental accreditation standards.

CONTENTS

NEPHROLOGY/UROLOGY

NEUROLOGY

ORTHOPEDICS

PULMONARY

RHEUMATOLOGY

CONTRIBUTORS

Charles Chiu, MD
University of California, San Francisco, Resident in Internal Medicine

Kalpita Shah, PA-C
University of Texas Medical Branch, Galveston, Class of 2000

Mae Sheikh-Ali, MD
University of Damascus, Syria, Class of 1999

Pourya M.Ghazi, MD
Senior Fellow, Department of Laboratory Medicine, University of Washington, Seattle

Sonal Shah, MD
Ross University, Class of 2000

Vaneesh Soni
University of Michigan, Ann Arbor, Class of 2006

Vipal Soni, MD
UCLA School of Medicine, Class of 1999

Zubin Damania, MD
University of California, San Francisco, Class of 1999

Faculty Reviewer

Thomas A. Blackwell, MD
Program Director, Program in Internal Medicine
University of Texas Medical Branch, Galveston

Vishal Pall, MD, MPH
Internist and Preventive Medicine Specialist
Government Medical College, Chandigarh - Panjab University – India, Class of 1997
Graduate School of Biomedical Sciences at UTMB Galveston, MPH Class of 2004

ACKNOWLEDGMENTS

Throughout the production of this book, we have had the support of many friends and colleagues. Special thanks to our support team including Andrea Fellows, Anastasia Anderson, Srishti Gupta, Anu Gupta, Mona Pall, Jonathan Kirsch, and Chirag Amin. For prior contributions we thank Gianni Le Nguyen, Tarun Mathur, Alex Grimm, Sonia Santos, and Elizabeth Sanders.

For submitting comments, corrections, editing, proofreading, and assistance across all of the vignette titles in all editions, we collectively thank:

Tara Adamovich, Carolyn Alexander, Kris Alden, Henry E. Aryan, Lynman Bacolor, Natalie Barteneva, Dean Bartholomew, Debashish Behera, Sumit Bhatia, Sanjay Bindra, Dave Brinton, Julianne Brown, Alexander Brownie, Tamara Callahan, David Canes, Bryan Casey, Aaron Caughey, Hebert Chen, Jonathan Cheng, Arnold Cheung, Arnold Chin, Simion Chiosea, Yoon Cho, Samuel Chung, Gretchen Conant, Vladimir Coric, Christopher Cosgrove, Ronald Cowan, Karekin R. Cunningham, A. Sean Dalley, Rama Dandamudi, Sunit Das, Ryan Armando Dave, John David, Emmanuel de la Cruz, Robert DeMello, Navneet Dhillon, Sharmila Dissanaike, David Donson, Adolf Etchegaray, Alea Eusebio, Priscilla A. Frase, David Frenz, Kristin Gaumer, Yohannes Gebreegziabher, Anil Gehi, Tony George, L.M. Gotanco, Parul Goyal, Alex Grimm, Rajeev Gupta, Ahmad Halim, Sue Hall, David Hasselbacher, Tamra Heimert, Michelle Higley, Dan Hoit, Eric Jackson, Tim Jackson, Sundar Jayaraman, Pei-Ni Jone, Aarchan Joshi, Rajni K. Jutla, Faiyaz Kapadi, Seth Karp, Aaron S. Kesselheim, Sana Khan, Andrew Pin-wei Ko, Francis Kong, Paul Konitzky, Warren S. Krackov, Benjamin H.S. Lau, Ann LaCasce, Connie Lee, Scott Lee, Guillermo Lehmann, Kevin Leung, Paul Levett, Warren Levinson, Eric Ley, Ken Lin, Pavel Lobanov, J. Mark Maddox, Aram Mardian, Samir Mehta, Gil Melmed, Joe Messina, Robert Mosca, Michael Murphy, Vivek Nandkarni, Siva Naraynan, Carvell Nguyen, Linh Nguyen, Deanna Nobleza, Craig Nodurft, George Noumi, Darin T. Okuda, Adam L. Palance, Paul Pamphrus, Jinha Park, Shalin Patel, Sonny Patel, Ricardo Pietrobon, Riva L. Rahl, Aashita Randeria, Rachan Reddy, Beatriu Reig, Marilou Reyes, Jeremy Richmon, Tai Roe, Rick Roller, Rajiv Roy, Diego Ruiz, Anthony Russell, Sanjay Sahgal, Urmimala Sarkar, John Schilling, Isabell Schmitt, Daren Schuhmacher, Sonal Shah, Edie Shen, Justin Smith, John Stulak, Lillian Su, Julie Sundaram, Rita Suri, Seth Sweetser, Antonio Talayero, Merita Tan, Mark Tanaka, Eric Taylor, Jess Thompson, Indi Trehan, Raymond Turner, Okafo Uchenna, Eric Uyguanco, Richa Varma, John Wages, Alan Wang, Eunice Wang, Andy Weiss, Amy Williams, Brian Yang, Hany Zaky, Ashraf Zaman, and David Zipf.

Please let us know if your name has been missed or misspelled and we will be happy to make the update in the next edition.

For generously contributing images to the entire Underground Clinical Vignette Step 2 series, we collectively thank the staff at Blackwell Publishing in Oxford, Boston, and Berlin as well as:

- Alfred Cuschieri, Thomas P.J. Hennessy, Roger M. Greenhalgh, David I. Rowley, Pierce A. Grace (Clinical Surgery, © 1996 Blackwell Science), Figures 13.23, 13.35b, 13.51, 15.13, 15.2.

- Berg D. Advanced Clinical Skills and Physical Diagnosis. Blackwell Science Ltd., 1999. Figures 7.10, 7.12, 7.13, 7.2, 7.3, 7.7, 7.8, 7.9, 8.1, 8.2, 8.4, 8.5, 9.2, 10.2, 11.3, 11.5, 12.6.

- John Axford (Medicine, © 1996 Blackwell Science), Figures f3.10, 2.103a, 2.110b, 3.20a, 3.20b, 3.25b, 3.38a, 5.9Bi, 5.9Bii, 6.41a, 6.41b, 6.74b, 6.74c, 7.78ai, 7.78aii, 7.78b, 8.47b, 9.9e, f3.17, f3.36, f3.37, f5.27, f5.28, f5.45a, f5.48, f5.49a, f5.50, f5.65a, f5.67, f5.68, f8.27a, 10.120b, 11.63b, 11.63c, 11.68a, 11.68b, 11.68c, 12.37a, 12.37b.

- Peter Armstrong, Martin L. Wastie (Diagnostic Imaging, 4th Edition, © 1998 Blackwell Science), Figures 2.100, 2.108d, 2.109, 2.11, 2.112, 2.121, 2.122, 2.13, 2.1ba, 2.1bb, 2.36, 2.53, 2.54, 2.69a, 2.71, 2.80a, 2.81b, 2.82, 2.84a, 2.84b, 2.88, 2.89a, 2.89b, 2.90b, 2.94a, 2.94b, 2.96, 2.97, 2.98a, 2.98c, 3.11, 3.19, 3.20, 3.21, 3.22, 3.28, 3.30, 3.34, 3.35b, 3.35c, 3.36, 4.7, 4.8, 4.9, 5.29, 5.33, 5.58, 5.62, 5.63, 5.64, 5.65b, 5.66a, 5.66b, 5.69, 5.71, 5.75, 5.8, 5.9, 6.17a, 6.17b, 6.25, 6.28, 6.29c, 6.30, 7.13, 7.17a, 7.45a, 7.45b, 7.46, 7.50, 7.52, 7.53a, 7.57a, 7.58, 8.7a, 8.7b, 8.7c, 8.86, 8.8a, 8.96, 8.9a, 9.17a, 9.17b, 10.13a, 10.13b, 10.14a, 10.14b, 10.14c, 10.17a, 10.17b, 11.16b, 11.17a, 11.17b, 11.19, 11.23, 11.24, 11.2b, 11.2d, 11.30a, 11.30b, 12.12, 12.15, 12.18, 12.19, 12.3, 12.4, 12.8a, 12.8b, 13.13a, 13.18, 13.18a, 13.20, 13.22a, 13.22b, 13.29, 14.14a, 14.5, 14.6a, 15.25b, 15.29b, 15.31, 15.37, 17.4.

- N.C. Hughes-Jones, S.N. Wickramasinghe (Lecture Notes On: Haematology, 6th Edition, © 1996 Blackwell Science), Figures 2.1b, 2.2a, 3.14, 3.8, 4.3, 5.2b, 5.5a, 5.8, 7.1, 7.2, 7.3, 7.5, 8.1, 10.5b, 10.6, 11.1, plate 29, plate 34, plate 44, plate 45, plate 48, plate 5, plate 42.

- Thomas Grumme, Wolfgang Kluge, Konrad Kretzschmar, Andreas Roesler (Cerebral and Spinal Computed Tomography, 3rd Edition, © 1998 Blackwell Science), Figures 16.2b, 16.3, 16.6a, 17.1a, 18.1c, 18.5, 41.3c, 41.3d, 44.3, 46.8, 47.7, 48.2, 48.6a, 53.5, 55.2a, 55.2c, 56.2b, 57.1, 61.3a, 61.3b, 63.1a, 64.3a, 65.3c, 66.3b, 67.6, 70.1a, 70.3, 81.2a, 81.4, 82.2, 82.3, 84.6.

- P.R. Patel (Lecture Notes On: Radiology, © 1998 Blackwell Science), Figures 2.15, 2.16, 2.25, 2.26, 2.30, 2.31, 2.33, 2.36, 3.11, 3.16, 3.19, 3.4, 3.7, 4.19, 4.20, 4.38, 4.44, 4.45, 4.46, 4.47, 4.49, 4.5, 5.14, 5.6, 6.18, 6.19, 6.20, 6.21, 6.22, 6.31a, 6.31b, 7.18, 7.19, 7.21, 7.22, 7.32, 7.34, 7.41, 7.46a, 7.46b, 7.48, 7.49, 7.9, 8.2, 8.3, 8.4, 8.5, 8.8, 8.9, 9.12, 9.2, 9.3, 9.8, 9.9, 10.11, 10.16, 10.5.

- Ramsay Vallance (An Atlas of Diagnostic Radiology in Gastroenterology, © 1999 Blackwell Science), Figures 1.22, 2.57, 2.27, 2.55a, 2.58, 2.59.

HOW TO USE THIS BOOK

This series was originally developed to address the increasing number of clinical vignette questions on medical examinations, including the USMLE Step 1 and Step 2.

Each UCV 2 book uses a series of approximately 50 "supra-prototypical" cases as a way to condense testable facts and associations. The clinical vignettes in this series are designed to give added emphasis to pathogenesis, epidemiology, management, and complications. They also contain relevant extensive B/W imaging plates within each book. Additionally, each UCV 2 book contains approximately 30 to 60 MiniCases that focus on presenting only the key facts for that disease in a tightly edited fashion. Although each case tends to present all the signs, symptoms, and diagnostic findings for a particular illness, **patients generally will not present with such a "complete" picture either clinically or on a medical examination.** Cases are not meant to simulate a potential real patient or an exam vignette. **All the boldfaced "buzzwords" are for learning purposes** and are not necessarily expected to be found in any one patient with the disease.

Definitions of selected important terms are placed within the vignettes in (small caps) in parentheses. Other parenthetical remarks often refer to the pathophysiology or mechanism of disease. The format should also help students learn to present cases succinctly during oral "bullet" presentations on clinical rotations. The cases are meant to serve as a condensed review, not as a primary reference. The information provided in this book has been prepared with a great deal of thought and careful research. This book should not, however, be considered as your sole source of information. Corrections, suggestions, and submissions of new cases are encouraged and will be acknowledged and incorporated when appropriate in future editions.

We hope that you find the *Blackwell Underground Clinical Vignettes* series informative and useful. We welcome feedback and suggestions you have about this book, or any published by Blackwell Publishing.

Please e-mail us at medfeedback@bos.blackwellpublishing.com.

ABBREVIATIONS

A-a	alveolar-arterial (oxygen gradient)
AAA	abdominal aortic aneurysm
ABCs	airway, breathing, circulation
ABGs	arterial blood gases
ABPA	allergic bronchopulmonary aspergillosis
ABVD	Adriamycin, bleomycin, vinblastine, dacarbazine (chemotherapy)
ACE	angiotensin-converting enzyme
ACTH	adrenocorticotropic hormone
ADA	adenosine deaminase, American Diabetic Association
ADH	antidiuretic hormone
ADHD	attention-deficit hyperactivity disorder
AED	automatic external defibrillator
AFP	α-fetoprotein
AI	aortic insufficiency
AICD	automatic internal cardiac defibrillator
AIDS	acquired immunodeficiency syndrome
ALL	acute lymphocytic leukemia
ALS	amyotrophic lateral sclerosis
ALT	alanine aminotransferase
AML	acute myelogenous leukemia
AMP	adenosine monophosphate
ANA	antinuclear antibody
ANCA	antineutrophil cytoplasmic antibody
Angio	angiography
AP	anteroposterior
aPTT	activated partial thromboplastin time
ARDS	adult respiratory distress syndrome
ARF	acute renal failure
AS	ankylosing spondylitis
ASA	acetylsalicylic acid
5-ASA	5-aminosalicylic acid
ASD	atrial septal defect
ASO	antistreptolysin O
AST	aspartate aminotransferase
ATLS	Advanced Trauma Life Support (protocol)
ATN	acute tubular necrosis
ATPase	adenosine triphosphatase
ATRA	all-*trans*-retinoic acid
AV	arteriovenous, atrioventricular
AVPD	avoidant personality disorder
AXR	abdominal x-ray
AZT	azidothymidine (zidovudine)
BCG	bacille Calmette-Guérin
BE	barium enema
BP	blood pressure

BPD	borderline personality disorder
BPH	benign prostatic hypertrophy
BPK	B-cell progenitor kinase
BPM	beats per minute
BUN	blood urea nitrogen
CAA	cerebral amyloid angiopathy
CABG	coronary artery bypass grafting
CAD	coronary artery disease
CALLA	common acute lymphoblastic leukemia antigen
C-ANCA	cytoplasmic antineutrophil cytoplasmic antibody
CAO	chronic airway obstruction
CAP	community-acquired pneumonia
CBC	complete blood count
CBD	common bile duct
CBT	cognitive behavioral therapy
CCU	cardiac care unit
CD	cluster of differentiation
CDC	Centers for Disease Control
CEA	carcinoembryonic antigen
CF	cystic fibrosis
CFTR	cystic fibrosis transmembrane regulator
CFU	colony-forming unit
CHF	congestive heart failure
CJD	Creutzfeldt–Jakob disease
CK	creatine kinase
CK-MB	creatine kinase, MB fraction
CLL	chronic lymphocytic leukemia
CML	chronic myelogenous leukemia
CMV	cytomegalovirus
CN	cranial nerve
CNS	central nervous system
CO	cardiac output
COPD	chronic obstructive pulmonary disease
CPAP	continuous positive airway pressure
CPK	creatine phosphokinase
CPR	cardiopulmonary resuscitation
CRP	C-reactive protein
CSF	cerebrospinal fluid
CT	computed tomography
CVA	cerebrovascular accident
CXR	chest x-ray
D&C	dilatation and curettage
DAF	decay-accelerating factor
DC	direct current
DEXA	dual-energy x-ray absorptiometry

DHEA	dehydroepiandrosterone
DIC	disseminated intravascular coagulation
DIP	distal interphalangeal (joint)
DKA	diabetic ketoacidosis
DL_{CO}	diffusing capacity of carbon monoxide
DM	diabetes mellitus
DMD	Duchenne's muscular dystrophy
DNA	deoxyribonucleic acid
DNase	deoxyribonuclease
dsDNA	double-stranded DNA
DTP	diphtheria, tetanus, pertussis (vaccine)
DTRs	deep tendon reflexes
DTs	delirium tremens
DUB	dysfunctional uterine bleeding
DVT	deep venous thrombosis
EBV	Epstein–Barr virus
ECG	electrocardiography
Echo	echocardiography
ECMO	extracorporeal membrane oxygenation
EDTA	ethylenediamine tetraacetic acid
EEG	electroencephalography
EF	ejection fraction
EGD	esophagogastroduodenoscopy
E:I	expiratory-to-inspiratory (ratio)
ELISA	enzyme-linked immunosorbent assay
EM	electron microscopy
EMG	electromyography
ER	emergency room
ERCP	endoscopic retrograde cholangiopancreatography
ESR	erythrocyte sedimentation rate
EtOH	ethanol
FDA	Food and Drug Administration
Fe_{Na}	fractional excretion of sodium
FEV_1	forced expiratory volume in 1 second
FIGO	International Federation of Gynecology and Obstetrics (classification)
FIo_2	fraction of inspired oxygen
FNA	fine-needle aspiration
FRC	functional residual capacity
FSH	follicle-stimulating hormone
FTA	fluorescent treponemal antibody
FTA-ABS	fluorescent treponemal antibody absorption test
5-FU	5-fluorouracil
FVC	forced vital capacity
G6PD	glucose-6-phosphate dehydrogenase
GA	gestational age

GABA	gamma-aminobutyric acid
GABHS	group A β-hemolytic streptococcus
GAD	generalized anxiety disorder
GBM	glomerular basement membrane
G-CSF	granulocyte colony-stimulating factor
GERD	gastroesophageal reflux disease
GFR	glomerular filtration rate
GGT	gamma-glutamyltransferase
GI	gastrointestinal
GnRH	gonadotropin-releasing hormone
GU	genitourinary
HAV	hepatitis A virus
Hb	hemoglobin
HBcAg	hepatitis B core antigen
HBsAg	hepatitis B surface antigen
HBV	hepatitis B virus
hCG	human chorionic gonadotropin
HCl	hydrogen chloride
HCO$_3$	bicarbonate
Hct	hematocrit
HCV	hepatitis C virus
HDL	high-density lipoprotein
HEENT	head, eyes, ears, nose, and throat
HELLP	hemolysis, elevated liver enzymes, low platelets (syndrome)
HEV	hepatitis E virus
HGPRT	hypoxanthine-guanine phosphoribosyltransferase
HHV	human herpesvirus
5-HIAA	5-hydroxyindoleacetic acid
HIDA	hepato-iminodiacetic acid (scan)
HIV	human immunodeficiency virus
HLA	human leukocyte antigen
HPF	high-power field
HPI	history of present illness
HPV	human papillomavirus
HR	heart rate
HRCT	high-resolution computed tomography
HS	hereditary spherocytosis
HSG	hysterosalpingography
HSV	herpes simplex virus
HUS	hemolytic-uremic syndrome
IABC	intra-aortic balloon counterpulsation
ICA	internal carotid artery
ICD	implantable cardiac defibrillator
ICP	intracranial pressure
ICU	intensive care unit

ID/CC	identification and chief complaint
IDDM	insulin-dependent diabetes mellitus
IE	infectious endocarditis
IFA	immunofluorescent antibody
Ig	immunoglobulin
IL	interleukin
IM	infectious mononucleosis, intramuscular
INH	isoniazid
INR	International Normalized Ratio
123-ISS	iodine-123-labeled somatostatin
IUD	intrauterine device
IUGR	intrauterine growth retardation
IV	intravenous
IVC	inferior vena cava
IVIG	intravenous immunoglobulin
IVP	intravenous pyelography
JRA	juvenile rheumatoid arthritis
JVD	jugular venous distention
JVP	jugular venous pressure
KOH	potassium hydroxide
KS	Kaposi's sarcoma
KUB	kidney, ureter, bladder
LA	left atrium
LAMB	lentigines, atrial myxoma, blue nevi (syndrome)
LD	Leishman-Donovan (body)
LDH	lactate dehydrogenase
LDL	low-density lipoprotein
LES	lower esophageal sphincter
LFTs	liver function tests
LH	luteinizing hormone
LHRH	luteinizing hormone–releasing hormone
LKM	liver-kidney microsomal (antibody)
LMN	lower motor neuron
LP	lumbar puncture
L/S	lecithin-to-sphingomyelin (ratio)
LSD	lysergic acid diethylamide
LV	left ventricle, left ventricular
LVH	left ventricular hypertrophy
Lytes	electrolytes
Mammo	mammography
MAO	monoamine oxidase (inhibitor)
MAP	mean arterial pressure
MCA	middle cerebral artery
MCHC	mean corpuscular hemoglobin concentration
MCP	metacarpophalangeal (joint)

MCV	mean corpuscular volume
MDMA	3,4-methylene-dioxymethamphetamine ("Ecstasy")
MEN	multiple endocrine neoplasia
MGUS	monoclonal gammopathy of undetermined origin
MHC	major histocompatibility complex
MI	myocardial infarction
MIBG	metaiodobenzylguanidine
MMR	measles, mumps, rubella (vaccine)
MPTP	1-methyl-4-phenyl-tetrahydropyridine
MR	magnetic resonance (imaging)
mRNA	messenger ribonucleic acid
MRSA	methicillin-resistant *Staphylococcus aureus*
MS	multiple sclerosis
MTP	metatarsophalangeal (joint)
MuSK	muscle-specific kinase
MVA	motor vehicle accident
NADPH	reduced nicotinamide adenine dinucleotide phosphate
NAME	nevi, atrial myxoma, myxoid neurofibroma, ephilides (syndrome)
NG	nasogastric
NIDDM	non-insulin-dependent diabetes mellitus
NMDA	N-methyl-D-aspartate
NPO	nil per os (nothing by mouth)
NSAID	nonsteroidal anti-inflammatory drug
Nuc	nuclear medicine
OCD	obsessive-compulsive disorder
OCP	oral contraceptive pill
OCPD	obsessive-compulsive personality disorder
17-OHP	17-hydroxyprogesterone
OPC	organophosphate and carbamate
OS	opening snap
OTC	over the counter
PA	posteroanterior
2-PAM	pralidoxime
P-ANCA	perinuclear antineutrophil cytoplasmic antibody
Pa_{O_2}	partial pressure of oxygen
PAS	periodic acid Schiff
PBS	peripheral blood smear
P_{CO_2}	partial pressure of carbon dioxide
PCOD	polycystic ovary disease
PCP	phencyclidine
PCR	polymerase chain reaction
PCV	polycythemia vera
PDA	patent ductus arteriosus
PE	physical exam
PEEP	positive end-expiratory pressure

PET	positron emission tomography
PFTs	pulmonary function tests
PID	pelvic inflammatory disease
PIP	proximal interphalangeal (joint)
PKU	phenylketonuria
PMI	point of maximal impulse
PMN	polymorphonuclear (leukocyte)
PO	per os (by mouth)
Po_2	partial pressure of oxygen
PPD	purified protein derivative
PROM	premature rupture of membranes
PRPP	phosphoribosyl pyrophosphate
PSA	prostate-specific antigen
PT	prothrombin time
PTE	pulmonary thromboembolism
PTH	parathyroid hormone
PTSD	post-traumatic stress disorder
PTT	partial thromboplastin time
RA	rheumatoid arthritis, right atrial
RBC	red blood cell
RDW	red-cell distribution width
REM	rapid eye movement
RF	rheumatoid factor
RhoGAM	Rh immune globulin
RNA	ribonucleic acid
RPR	rapid plasma reagin
RR	respiratory rate
RS	Reed-Sternberg (cell)
RSV	respiratory syncytial virus
RTA	renal tubular acidosis
RUQ	right upper quadrant
RV	residual volume, right ventricle, right ventricular
RVH	right ventricular hypertrophy
SA	sinoatrial
SAH	subarachnoid hemorrhage
Sao_2	oxygen saturation in arterial blood
SBE	subacute bacterial endocarditis
SBFT	small bowel follow-through
SC	subcutaneous
SCC	squamous cell carcinoma
SIADH	syndrome of inappropriate secretion of antidiuretic hormone
SIDS	sudden infant death syndrome
SLE	systemic lupus erythematosus
SMA	smooth muscle antibody
SSPE	subacute sclerosing panencephalitis

SSRI	selective serotonin reuptake inhibitor
STD	sexually transmitted disease
SZPD	schizoid personality disorder
T_3	triiodothyronine
T_4	thyroxine
TAB	therapeutic abortion
TB	tuberculosis
TBSA	total body surface area
TCA	tricyclic antidepressant
TCD	transcranial Doppler
TD	tardive dyskinesia
TENS	transcutaneous electrical nerve stimulation
TFTs	thyroid function tests
THC	*trans*-tetrahydrocannabinol
TIA	transient ischemic attack
TIBC	total iron-binding capacity
TIPS	transjugular intrahepatic portosystemic shunt
TLC	total lung capacity
TMJ	temporomandibular joint (syndrome)
TMP-SMX	trimethoprim-sulfamethoxazole
TNF	tumor necrosis factor
TNM	tumor, node, metastasis (staging)
ToRCH	*Toxoplasma*, rubella, CMV, herpes zoster
tPA	tissue plasminogen activator
TPO	thyroid peroxidase
TRAP	tartrate-resistant acid phosphatase
TRH	thyrotropin-releasing hormone
TSH	thyroid-stimulating hormone
TSS	toxic shock syndrome
TSST	toxic shock syndrome toxin
TTP	thrombotic thrombocytopenic purpura
TUBD	transurethral balloon dilatation
TUIP	transurethral incision of the prostate
TURP	transurethral resection of the prostate
UA	urinalysis
UGI	upper GI (series)
UMN	upper motor neuron
URI	upper respiratory infection
US	ultrasound
UTI	urinary tract infection
UV	ultraviolet
VCUG	voiding cystourethrogram
VDRL	Venereal Disease Research Laboratory
VF	ventricular fibrillation
VIN	vulvar intraepithelial neoplasia

VLDL	very low density lipoprotein
VMA	vanillylmandelic acid
V/Q	ventilation-perfusion (ratio)
VS	vital signs
VSD	ventricular septal defect
VT	ventricular tachycardia
vWF	von Willebrand factor
VZIG	varicella-zoster immune globulin
VZV	varicella-zoster virus
WAGR	Wilms' tumor, aniridia, ambiguous genitalia, mental retardation (syndrome)
WBC	white blood cell
WG	Wegener's granulomatosis
WPW	Wolff–Parkinson–White (syndrome)
XR	x-ray

ID/CC

A 68-year-old **white male** who works as a **farmer** complains of several discrete dry, rough, scaly lesions on his **forehead**.

HPI

He has worked **outdoors** for many years and has **never used sunscreen**. He states that he first noticed the lesions several months ago but adds that they are not painful unless he runs his fingers over them.

PE

VS: normal. PE: **fair-skinned** with **blond hair** and **blue eyes**; numerous small (< 1 cm), coarse, yellow-brown lesions with reddish tinge on forehead, ears, posterior neck, and dorsal aspect of hands (sun-exposed regions).

Labs

Skin biopsy shows **epidermal pleomorphic keratinocytes.**

Pathogenesis

Actinic or solar keratosis results from repeated and prolonged exposure to ultraviolet light (primarily UVB 290 to 320 nm), ionizing radiation, or polycyclic aromatic hydrocarbons and arsenicals, leading to damage to keratinocytes. Clonal expansion of mutated forms of the tumor suppressor gene p53 has been observed in cases of both actinic keratosis and squamous cell carcinoma, indicating that actinic keratosis is indeed a **premalignant lesion** that may be regarded as **squamous cell carcinoma in situ.**

Epidemiology

Actinic keratosis, like squamous cell carcinoma of the skin, occurs with increased frequency among **males**, individuals with a **light complexion**, those who **work outdoors**, people who frequent tanning salons, and individuals from Australia or the southwestern United States; the disease is rarely seen in blacks or East Indians. Immunosuppressed patients are also at increased risk.

Management

The initial treatment of uncomplicated lesions involves the **topical application of 5-FU and/or liquid nitrogen**. A **skin biopsy** may be necessary to rule out squamous cell carcinoma if evidence of ulceration or induration is present. Extensive skin involvement or evidence of nodular lesions requires **surgical excision**. Prevention primarily involves the use of **UVA/UVB sunscreens.**

Complications

Approximately 1 in 1,000 solar keratosis lesions will develop into invasive squamous cell carcinoma each year.

ID/CC   A 44-year-old male complains of **sore, scaly hands**.

HPI   The patient states that he has worked as a **bricklayer** (chronic exposure to chromate salts in cement) for the past 20 years. He adds that the condition of his hands has gradually worsened over the past year.

PE   VS: normal. PE: **bilateral hyperkeratosis, maceration, fissuring, and erosion of palms and proximal portion of each digit.**

Labs   Patch test elicits a local response at a distant site.

Pathogenesis   Contact dermatitis appears in two forms: **nonallergic** (caused by chemical irritation) and **allergic/eczematous (type IV hypersensitivity reaction to an antigen).** Acids and bases cause irritant contact dermatitis, while poison ivy and oak usually cause allergic contact dermatitis. Irritant contact dermatitis is concentration dependent and sharply marginated and does not require sensitization (unlike allergic contact dermatitis, which depends on sensitization). Chronic toxic or irritant dermatitis results from repeated exposure to agents that gradually erode the barrier function of the skin and ultimately elicit an inflammatory response.

Epidemiology   Occupational exposures play a crucial role in the etiology of contact dermatitis. Young children only infrequently present with allergic contact dermatitis, and black individuals appear to be less susceptible.

Management   Removal of offending agent; topical steroids. Additionally, one may drain large vesicles without uncovering them and apply wet dressings with Burow's solution every 3 hours for acute dermatitis.

CASE 3

ID/CC A 32-year-old man presents with an intensely **pruritic vesiculopapular** eruption limited to the extensor surfaces of his knees and elbows.

HPI The patient reports **repeated episodes** of the rash over the past few years. The first episode occurred at age 24.

PE VS: normal. PE: cardiopulmonary exam normal; pruritic vesiculopapular eruption on extensor surfaces of knees and elbows; remainder of exam normal.

Labs Direct immunofluorescence of normal perilesional skin demonstrates granular deposits of IgA in papillary dermis and along epidermal basement membrane zone; no circulating IgA.

Pathogenesis Dermatitis herpetiformis is an idiopathic autoimmune disease characterized by **granular deposits of IgA** in the papillary dermis and along the epidermal basement membrane zone with intensely pruritic, chronic vesiculopapular lesions symmetrically distributed over the extensor surfaces.

Epidemiology Greater than 90% of patients with dermatitis herpetiformis are **HLA-B8/DRw3 and HLA-DQw2 positive**. Almost all have associated, usually subclinical **gluten-sensitive enteropathy.**

Management Maintenance of a **gluten-free diet** may diminish outbreaks. **Dapsone** should be used in exacerbations.

ID/CC   A 23-year-old female presents to the clinic complaining of **painful, tender nodules on the anterior surface of her leg.**

HPI   She had a **fever** and **sore throat** prior to the appearance of the lesions. She also complains of an **aching pain in her ankles.**

PE   VS: **fever** (38.6°C). PE: **numerous deep red** (ERYTHEMATOUS), round lesions 3 to 20 cm in diameter that are poorly demarcated and located on lower legs bilaterally; palpable nodules that are indurated and tender.

Labs   ESR elevated; throat culture positive for group A β-hemolytic streptococci (GABHS).

Imaging   CXR: normal.

Pathogenesis Erythema nodosum is an acute inflammatory or immunologic disorder leading to a septal panniculitis in subcutaneous fat. It arises in **response to infectious agents** (e.g., GABHS, *Yersinia*, histoplasmosis, **coccidioidomycosis**, and tuberculosis), in **inflammatory conditions** such as sarcoidosis and **ulcerative colitis**, and in response to **drugs** such as sulfonamides and OCPs. Generally, the condition remits spontaneously within 6 weeks.

Epidemiology The most common cause of acute panniculitis. Patients are generally **female** (3:1) and **between the ages of 15 and 30.**

Management Treat the underlying cause and initiate supportive measures such as bed rest, decreased weight bearing, compressive bandages, and/or NSAIDs. In severe cases where infectious agents have been ruled out, prednisone may be administered.

Complications Complications are related to the underlying disease.

ID/CC

A 34-year-old **homosexual** male presents with unusual **purple-red, painless skin lesions** about the face and neck.

HPI

He also complains of shortness of breath and adds that he has had dull chest pain and a limited appetite and has **coughed up blood** on a few occasions (HEMOPTYSIS). He has been **HIV positive** for 6 years.

PE

VS: normal. PE: pallor; multiple mucocutaneous **purplish macules**; palpable abdominal masses and tenderness; generalized indurated lymphadenopathy; pedal edema.

Labs

CBC: anemia; thrombocytosis; lymphopenia. **CD4 lymphocyte count decreased** (155×10^6/L); biopsy of lesion reveals **proliferation of spindle cells, endothelial cells**, and extravasation of RBCs.

Imaging

CXR: bilateral lower lobe infiltrates obscure the margins of the mediastinum and diaphragm (finding suggestive of **pulmonary metastases**). Fiberoptic bronchoscopy and endoscopy for visualization and biopsy of other suspected Kaposi's sarcoma (KS) sites should be performed. Stage the tumor with a chest CT and bone scan.

Pathogenesis

KS is a **hemangiosarcoma** that may affect the skin, viscera, and mucous membranes. The lymph nodes, GI tract, and lungs are also commonly involved. KS is usually seen as an "opportunistic" neoplasm in HIV-positive homosexual men but may be seen during any stage of the infection. Etiologic associations include Kaposi's sarcoma-associated virus (HHV-8).

Epidemiology

KS in a male younger than 60 years is strongly suggestive of HIV infection. Ninety-six percent of AIDS-related cases occur in homosexual men. KS is rare in children and hemophiliacs with AIDS.

Management

Optimize control of HIV infection with effective antiretroviral therapy. Local therapy includes radiation therapy, intralesional vinblastine, cryotherapy and topical retinoids for cutaneous lesions, and **resection of isolated lung metastases**. Few AIDS patients with KS die as a result of this malignancy; thus, treatment regimens that suppress the immune system should be avoided. Treatment may be indicated for lesions that are associated with significant discomfort (e.g., those located over a joint), dysphagia (e.g., oropharyngeal lesions), or cosmetic problems (e.g., facial lesions). **Interferon** is useful in early disease. **Combination chemotherapy** with doxorubicin, etoposide, vinblastine, and bleomycin is warranted in aggressive KS. Prognosis is related to CD4 count and immune status.

Complications

Ulceration of the cutaneous lesion with subsequent infection is a common side effect of therapy; GI obstruction and hemorrhage may occur with internal lesions.

ID/CC An 18-year-old man presents with **scaly salmon-pink lesions** on the extensor surfaces of his elbows and knees.

HPI The patient is otherwise healthy.

PE VS: normal. PE: **erythematous papules and plaques** with silver scaling on extensor surfaces of elbows and knees; nail pitting of hands.

Labs Skin biopsy shows focal parakeratosis, hyperkeratosis, elongation and thickening of rete ridges, and thinning of epidermis above dermal papillae.

Pathogenesis Psoriasis is an idiopathic disease, perhaps autoimmune in origin, that is characterized by epidermal proliferation with **increased thickness of the stratum spinosum** (ACANTHOSIS), **retention of nuclei in the cells of the stratum corneum** (PARAKERATOSIS) and collections of neutrophils (MONRO'S MICROABSCESSES) within the stratum corneum; it most often involves the **extensor surfaces** of the elbows and knees, scalp, and sacral areas.

Epidemiology A common dermatologic disease. Thirty-five percent of patients have a family history of psoriasis.

Management Mild to moderate psoriasis can be treated with **topical corticosteroids**. **Keratolytic agents** (e.g., salicylic acid) can be used when marked hyperkeratosis is present. **Topical retinoids** or **tar compounds** may be beneficial when alternated with corticosteroids. Severe psoriasis should be treated **chemotherapeutically** (methotrexate, cyclosporin) and with **UV light**.

Complications Extensive disease can lead to **psoriatic arthritis**. Secondary bacterial infection may occur as well (pustular psoriasis).

ID/CC

A 74-year-old man with Parkinson's disease presents with a greasy, **scaly rash** that has spread from his scalp to his eyebrows, eyelids, and nasolabial folds.

HPI

The patient reports increased itching over the involved areas. He had been treated for severe dandruff in the past year.

PE

VS: normal. PE: bilateral, symmetrically distributed patches of greasy, erythematous scales localized to hair-covered areas of the head and nasolabial folds.

Pathogenesis

Seborrheic dermatitis is a common, chronic disorder characterized by **greasy scales** overlying erythematous plaques or patches. Lesions are most commonly located on the scalp (may be recognized as severe dandruff) but may also affect the eyebrows, eyelids, glabella, nasolabial folds, or ears. Although the condition is more frequently seen in patients with Parkinson's disease, cerebrovascular accident, or HIV, the majority of individuals with seborrheic dermatitis have no underlying disorder. Its etiology is thought to be an inflammatory reaction to the yeast *Pityrosporum*.

Epidemiology

May be evident in the first weeks of life, commonly affecting the scalp (CRADLE CAP). It is rarely seen in children after infancy but is evident again in adulthood. Affects approximately 3% of the general population.

Management

Treat the scalp with 2.5% selenium sulfide, zinc pyrithione, tar, salicylic acid, or ketoconazole shampoo. Apply **low-dose corticosteroids** or **ketoconazole** cream to the affected skin in severe cases.

TOP SECRET

ID/CC   A 63-year-old white male presents with a reddish nodule on the left side of his lip that has failed to heal for several months.

HPI   The patient reports a tendency to sunburn due to his fair skin. He had another lesion in the same location that was diagnosed as actinic keratosis almost 10 years ago. The present lesion is not painful or pruritic.

PE   VS: normal. PE: blond and fair-skinned; no acute distress; HEENT remarkable for 6.0- × 8.0-mm red, conical, hard nodule with ulceration on superior aspect of lower left lip margin.

Labs   Biopsy of lesion reveals invasion of dermis by sheets and islands of neoplastic epidermal cells, often with "keratin pearls."

Pathogenesis   Squamous cell carcinoma (SCC) is a malignant neoplasm of keratinizing epithelial cells. It may develop anywhere on the body but typically involves sun-damaged skin. Several premalignant forms should be noted, including actinic keratosis, actinic cheilitis, and Bowen's disease (may develop into SCC in 20% of cases).

Epidemiology   Nonmelanoma skin cancer is the most common cancer in the United States, with > 800,000 cases diagnosed each year; SCC accounts for approximately 20% of cases (basal cell carcinoma accounts for 70% to 80%). The causes are multifactorial, including cumulative exposure to UVB sunlight, male sex, older age, Celtic ancestry, fair complexion, tendency to sunburn, and outdoor occupation. As many as 45% of patients with renal transplants develop SCC within 10 years.

Management   Surgical excision is the mainstay of treatment; Mohs' microsurgery, radiation, and cryosurgery are alternate modalities. Metastases are treated with lymph node dissection, irradiation, or both. Because most cases are related to chronic UVB exposure, emphasis should be placed on prevention with regular use of sunscreens and protective clothing. Close follow-up for detection of recurrence, metastasis, or new cancers is indicated in all patients with a history of skin cancer.

Complications   SCC carries a low but significant malignant potential. Metastases occur in 5% to 10% of patients with cutaneous lesions, 11% of ear lesions, and 13% of lower lip lesions; the rate of metastasis is higher for cancers arising in burn scars, chronic ulcerations, genitalia, and recurrent tumors. Regional lymph nodes are the most common site of metastasis. The prognosis is poor in patients with metastatic disease.

ID/CC	An 18-year-old male presents with refractory **myopia** and **scoliosis**.
HPI	He complains that his schoolmates make fun of his **exceptionally long arms, fingers, and legs.**
PE	VS: normal. PE: slit-lamp exam shows **ectopia lentis** (lens dislocation); moderate **chest wall depression** (PECTUS EXCAVATUM); marked **scoliosis**; midsystolic click and soft 2/6 systolic murmur (mitral valve prolapse) audible at apex with radiation to axilla; aortic diastolic murmur (aortic insufficiency), limbs long and thin with **increased arm span**; moderate **arachnodactyly.**
Labs	Normal.
Imaging	Echo: **mitral valve prolapse** with mild mitral valve insufficiency and mild **aortic root dilatation** with mild aortic insufficiency.
Pathogenesis	Marfan's syndrome is an **autosomal-dominant** connective tissue disease that results from **a mutation in the fibrillin gene** (chromosome 15). Fibrillin is a 350-kDa glycoprotein that serves as a major component of elastin-associated microfibrils abundant in large blood vessels and the suspensory ligaments of the lens. **Cystic medial necrosis** of the aorta (predisposing to dissection) and **myxomatous cardiac valve** (usually aortic and mitral) disease are classical abnormalities.
Epidemiology	Occurs in 1 in 10,000 persons. Approximately 25% of patients have no affected parents; these are usually due to a new mutation. Affects both genders equally.
Management	**Regular ophthalmologic surveillance** (follow closely for visual acuity to prevent amblyopia and retinal detachment); **annual orthopedic consultation** to ensure early diagnosis of scoliosis; annual echocardiography to monitor aortic diameter and mitral valve function; **endocarditis prophylaxis.** Beta-adrenergic blockade to retard the rate of aortic dilatation; restrict significant physical activity to protect against aortic dissection. **Prophylactic replacement of the aortic root** with composite graft should be considered when the diameter approaches 50 to 55 mm (normal < 40 mm).
Complications	Mitral valve prolapse typically develops early in life and can result in mitral insufficiency (the most common cause of death in children); aortic root dilatation can result in aortic regurgitation, aortic dissection, or aortic rupture. **Ectopia lentis** is a central diagnostic feature that results in cataract formation, ocular globe elongation, and retinal detachment. **Spontaneous pneumothoraces** secondary to multiple thoracic cage deformities (pectus excavatum, scoliosis) as well as **inguinal and incisional hernias** are common. In untreated patients, mortality may result in the fourth or fifth decade due to aortic dissection or CHF secondary to aortic regurgitation.

GENETICS

ID/CC A 40-year-old **male** complains of high, intermittent, spiking **fever with chills, right upper quadrant abdominal pain**, malaise, anorexia, and nausea of 1 week's duration.

HPI He is a missionary who just returned from a 3-year stay in **rural South America**. Directed questioning reveals that he suffered from **diarrhea with blood and mucus** (DYSENTERY) as well as tenesmus on several occasions (due to intestinal amebiasis). He additionally reports a 4-kg weight loss over the past 2 months.

PE VS: **fever** (39.3°C); tachycardia (HR 110); normal BP. PE: pallor; slight jaundice; no lymphadenopathy; right lung field shows **diminished breath sounds and basilar rales**; soft tissue edema and shiny appearance over right upper quadrant with **marked, tender hepatomegaly**; no ascites, spider angiomata, or caput medusae.

Labs CBC: **anemia** (Hb 10.4); marked **leukocytosis** (18,350); **neutrophilia** (89%). Elevated ESR; **amebic trophozoites and ova in stool** (positivity rate is 10% to 30%); chocolate-colored ("anchovy sauce") pus obtained by needle aspiration of abscess does not show parasites (positivity rate is < 30%; amebae are confined to the periphery of lesion); positive complement fixation test reaction to *Entamoeba histolytica*.

Imaging [**Fig. 10A**] US, abdomen: a large hypoechoic mass (1) is seen in the liver in another patient; note the diaphragm (D) and kidney (K). [**Fig. 10B**] CT, abdomen: a different case in which two areas of low attenuation are seen in the right lobe of the liver. [**Fig. 10C**] XR, abdomen: an air-fluid level is seen in this right subphrenic abscess (the normal gastric bubble is seen on the left).

Pathogenesis Amebic abscess of the liver is a complication of intestinal infection with *Entamoeba histolytica*. A history of prior travel to an endemic area plus the triad of **fever, hepatomegaly**, and **right upper quadrant pain** are characteristics of hepatic amebic abscess.

Epidemiology The liver is the most common extraintestinal location of amebiasis; prior intestinal infection may be asymptomatic or may present as amebic dysentery. The abscess is usually **single** and more commonly presents in the posterosuperior surface of the **right lobe of the liver**. It shows a **male predominance**.

Management **Metronidazole** is the mainstay of therapy and is usually given with iodoquinol as a luminal amebicide. Dehydroemetine may be used for resistant cases and may be followed by chloroquine. Most abscesses will respond to medical therapy. Attempt **percutaneous aspiration/surgical drainage** for imminent rupture, large abscesses, location in the left lobe

continued

(danger of pericardial rupture), secondary bacterial infection, or failure of medical treatment. Rule out hydatidiform disease (ECHINOCOCCOSIS) before attempting aspiration.

Complications **Secondary pyogenic infection** is the most common complication. **Rupture** may be life-threatening. Involvement of the psoas and gluteus muscle, pararectal spaces, spleen, or brain may occur by contiguity or metastatic dissemination.

Figure 10A

Figure 10B

Figure 10C

ID/CC A 45-year-old man with bronchial **asthma** complains of a **productive cough.**

HPI He also complains of progressively increasing breathlessness with intermittent attacks of severe dyspnea. He notes the presence of **brownish plugs** in his sputum.

PE VS: **tachypnea** (RR 28). PE: mild respiratory distress; mild **cyanosis**; pallor; occasional rhonchi and wheezes heard bilaterally; **clubbing** of fingernails.

Labs CBC: **eosinophilia.** Skin testing reveals immediate reaction to *Aspergillus fumigatus*; serum IgG to *A. fumigatus* present; serum IgE elevated; sputum culture grows *A. fumigatus.*

Imaging CXR: branching, fingerlike shadows from mucoid impaction of dilated central bronchi involving the upper lobes (virtually pathognomonic).

Pathogenesis Allergic bronchopulmonary aspergillosis is characterized by preexisting asthma accompanied by eosinophilia, IgE antibody to *Aspergillus*, and fleeting finger-shaped pulmonary infiltrates on CXR.

Epidemiology Usually seen in atopic asthmatic individuals 20 to 40 years old.

Management Allergen avoidance along with symptomatic management with **corticosteroids** and treatment of underlying lung disease (bronchodilators) are indicated. Systemic **antifungal therapy is not effective** in endobronchial disease.

Complications *Aspergillus* may occasionally colonize a preexisting pulmonary cavity and produce an aspergilloma, which may be complicated by hemoptysis and should be treated by lobectomy. **Invasive aspergillosis** may occur in immune-compromised patients.

ID/CC	A 28-year-old male is brought to the ER complaining of sudden-onset **double vision**, hoarseness, **slurred speech**, and **difficulty swallowing** for the past few hours.
HPI	He also reports repeated vomiting and **symmetric weakness** of the extremities that has **progressed caudally**. Directed questioning reveals that he ate some **home-canned stew** yesterday.
PE	VS: **no fever**; postural hypotension. PE: **alert** but in acute distress; severe abdominal tenderness; bowel sounds depressed; ocular exam reveals **ptosis, dilated pupils sluggishly reacting to light**, and extraocular muscle paresis (type A may have no ocular signs); **DTRs depressed** in proportion to weakness.
Labs	Blood positive for *Clostridium botulinum* toxin. PFTs: spirometry reveals normal vital capacity (to rule out respiratory muscle weakness).
Pathogenesis	Botulism is an acute **descending paralytic disease** that **begins in the cranial nerves** and **descends caudally** to affect the extremities (without sensory deficits). Botulinum toxin **blocks acetylcholine release** in motor nerve terminals, resulting in a **flaccid paralysis**. Autonomic nerve endings may also be affected, resulting in dry mouth, constipation, or urine retention. Cases may be classified as **food-borne** botulism (derived from contaminated food), **wound** botulism (from localized toxin production), **infant** botulism (ingestion and/or gut production in infants), **adult-infant** botulism (similar to infants, but affecting older children and adults), or indeterminate. **Botulism should be considered only in afebrile, oriented patients who have a descending paralysis.**
Epidemiology	Botulism occurs worldwide. Of the eight known types of *C. botulinum* toxins (types A–G), types A, B, and E commonly cause disease in humans. Food-borne illness is associated with **home-canned vegetables, fruit, and condiments** (infant poisoning is associated with contaminated honey). This type of botulism occurs when contaminated food is preserved with **spores** or when food is not heated to a temperature that destroys the **toxin**.
Management	**Equine antitoxin** emergently while monitoring the patient for anaphylaxis and serum sickness. Emetic and gastric lavage may be useful if ingestion of contaminated food is recent. Infant botulism is not helped by antibiotics. Antibiotics that act at the neuromuscular junctions **(aminoglycosides) should be avoided**. Monitor spirometry, pulse oximetry, and ABGs to guard against **respiratory failure**. If vital capacity falls < 30%, intubation and **mechanical ventilation** are required, especially if paralysis, hypercarbia, and hypoxemia are progressing.
Complications	Fatalities from botulism poisoning are low due to the availability of respiratory support. Artificial respiration may be required for weeks in severe cases, and residual autonomic dysfunction may be observed.

INFECTIOUS DISEASE

ID/CC

A 35-year-old male with **AIDS** complains of **diminution of vision** in his right eye.

HPI

The patient states that he sees **floaters** and acknowledges a recent **fever**.

PE

VS: **fever** (38.6°C). PE: funduscopic exam demonstrates **perivascular hemorrhagic exudates** and necrotic areas in right eye; decreased visual acuity.

Labs

CD4 count < 50.

Pathogenesis

CMV retinitis arises following **reactivation of a latent infection**, most commonly in AIDS patients with CD4 counts < 100. It causes progressive **necrotizing retinitis** that eventually leads to blindness.

Epidemiology

CMV is common; > 50% of adults have antibodies to the virus, and > 90% of homosexual men have **latent infections**. CMV retinitis is the most common opportunistic eye infection in HIV patients.

Management

Treatment may be local (to the affected eye alone), systemic, or a combination of both. Treatment options include IV ganciclovir, foscarnet, and cidofovir; oral ganciclovir; intravitreous injection of ganciclovir, foscarnet, and fomivirsen; and surgically implanted slow-release ganciclovir devices.

Complications

Retinal detachment and blindness, line sepsis from IV drug administration, and CMV involvement of the contralateral eye or other end-organ involvement (pneumonitis, colitis, encephalitis).

ID/CC

A 40-year-old male complains of **fever, cough, arthralgias**, and generalized malaise of 2 days' duration.

HPI

He also complains of left-sided pleuritic chest pain and mentions that he recently noticed a few **painful red lesions** on his shins. Three days ago he returned from a trip to the **southwestern United States**.

PE

VS: fever (38.9°C); tachypnea. PE: rales heard over left lower lobe; multiple tender **erythematous nodules** over both shins (ERYTHEMA NODOSUM); movements at large joints (knees and ankles) restricted by pain.

Labs

CBC/PBS: eosinophilia. *Coccidioides immitis* **spherules seen on sputum stain; coccidioidin skin test positive** (5-mm area of induration 48 hours after intradermal injection of coccidioidin).

Imaging

CXR: left lower lobe consolidation with hilar adenopathy.

Pathogenesis

The causative agent is *Coccidioides immitis*, a dimorphic fungus that grows in its natural soil habitat and on routine culture as a mold composed of **septate hyphae-bearing arthrospores**. The arthrospores are detached and swept into an aerosol that can easily be inhaled. Within the host, the highly infectious arthrospores mature into **spherules, the definitive tissue pathogen**. The spectrum of the disease varies from a primary pulmonary infection (whose severity varies from a mild influenza-like illness to severe pneumonitis) to a disseminated systemic form (more frequent in blacks and in pregnant or immune-compromised patients).

Epidemiology

The natural habitat of *C. immitis* is the desert soil of parts of California (e.g., **San Joaquin Valley**), southern Arizona, Utah, New Mexico, Nevada, southwestern Texas, Mexico, and Central and South America. The recent increase in reported cases has been largely due to the increased prevalence of AIDS, recent dust storms and earthquakes, and increased physician recognition of the disease. **Human-to-human transmission does not occur.**

Management

Mild to moderate disease **usually resolves without treatment**. **Amphotericin B** is the treatment of choice for critically ill patients; follow with oral **itraconazole** or **ketoconazole** for long-term suppression in HIV-positive and immune-compromised patients. Surgery may be necessary for chronic and progressive pulmonary lesions.

Complications

Disseminated disease; chronic meningitis; skin lesions (maculopapular rash).

INFECTIOUS DISEASE

ID/CC	A 35-year-old female presents with **delirium**.
HPI	She suddenly developed an **influenza-like syndrome approximately 1 week ago**. It has included **fever, chills, headaches, rigors, malaise, and cough**. Over the last several days, she has also developed a **truncal rash** and has become less coherent.
PE	VS: fever (38.7°C). PE: disoriented; **prominent maculopapular rash on trunk with several incipient lesions on extremities**; coarse breath sounds and rales bilaterally.
Labs	CBC: elevated WBC; normal hemoglobin, hematocrit, and platelets. **Weil-Felix test positive for antirickettsial antibodies**.
Imaging	CXR: bilateral patchy pulmonary infiltrates.
Pathogenesis	Epidemic typhus is caused by *Rickettsia prowazekii*, an obligate intracellular parasite that is **transmitted to humans by the body louse**. The disease begins when an infected individual is bitten by a louse, which ingests the rickettsial organism with the blood meal. The organism then multiplies in the gut of the louse. While biting another individual, the louse feces are excreted with *R. prowazekii*. The individual scratches, causing autoinoculation. One to three weeks after infection, the newly infected individual develops a flulike illness followed by a rash and signs of meningoencephalitis 5 to 9 days later.
Epidemiology	Epidemic typhus typically arises in times and places with **poor sanitation, crowding**, and **infrequent bathing**. Consequently, it has not been seen in the United States in more than 50 years. Among individuals who do contract the disease and are untreated, the mortality rate ranges from 10% to 60% and increases with age.
Management	**Tetracycline** (chloramphenicol second line). Prophylaxis depends on good **personal hygiene** and use of protective clothing in regions where typhus is prevalent. An inactivated vaccine of *R. prowazekii* is available abroad and for military personnel.
Complications	Myocarditis, intestinal hemorrhage, jaundice, renal insufficiency, vasculitis and thrombosis, and meningoencephalitis leading to delirium, coma, and death.

CASE 16

ID/CC

A 19-year-old male college student complains of urinary urgency and **painful urination** (DYSURIA) for the past 3 days.

HPI

He also complains of painful **swelling of the left side of his scrotum** (due to epididymitis). He notes that his underwear has been stained with a thick, greenish, purulent urethral discharge that is more profuse in the morning. He had **unprotected sex** during spring break **1 week ago** with a local striptease dancer.

PE

VS: normal. PE: erythema and swelling of urethral meatus with a thick, greenish-yellow, purulent discharge expressed; **left epididymis swollen, hard, and exquisitely tender**; normal prostate.

Labs

CBC: leukocytosis (11,500); 75% neutrophils. Gram stain of discharge shows **abundant PMNs** with **intracellular gram-negative diplococci**; culture in Thayer–Martin medium grows *Neisseria gonorrhoeae*; VDRL negative.

Pathogenesis

Gonorrhea is an STD caused by *Neisseria gonorrhoeae*, an oxidase-positive, gram-negative, intracellular diplococcus.

Epidemiology

Gonorrhea is a prevalent communicable disease in the United States. Its **incubation period varies from 2 to 10 days**; females are often asymptomatic carriers.

Management

Antibiotic therapy for uncomplicated disease consists of **ceftriaxone** (first line). Treatment should be followed by doxycycline or azithromycin owing to the **possibility of coexisting infection with** *Chlamydia trachomatis*. Complicated disease requires IV penicillin. **Treatment of sexual partners** is essential.

Complications

Patients may develop severe GU involvement and dissemination to virtually any organ or structure. Notable complications include PID with resultant sterility, **septic monoarthritis**, perihepatitis (FITZ–HUGH–CURTIS SYNDROME), and **ophthalmia neonatorum** in newborns.

INFECTIOUS DISEASE

TOP SECRET

ID/CC   A 27-year-old **sexually active** male presents with **painful penile lesions.**

HPI   The patient also complains of **burning, itching,** and a **tingling sensation.** The lesions have progressed from erythematous to vesicular to ulcerated.

PE   VS: low-grade fever (38.4°C). PE: numerous **vesicular and ulcerated lesions on shaft of penis; inguinal lymphadenopathy.**

Labs   **Tzanck smear with multinucleated giant cells.**

Pathogenesis   The causative agent is HSV-2; usually acquired and transmitted through sexual or perinatal contact. The virus replicates at the site of infection before migrating up neurons and becoming **latent in the sensory ganglia (trigeminal and lumbosacral)**; exposure to sunlight or UV light, immunosuppression, infections, fever, stress, hormonal changes, trauma, and depression may cause reactivation. HSV-2 causes genital herpes, neonatal herpes, and aseptic meningitis.

Epidemiology   One of the most common sexually transmitted infections.

Management   **Antiviral therapy** (e.g., **acyclovir,** ganciclovir) for primary infections and to suppress genital recurrences. Foscarnet (IV) may be given for acyclovir-resistant cases or immune-compromised patients with systemic disease. Encourage prevention via latex condom use and cautious interpersonal contact with patients harboring active lesions.

Complications   HSV-1 is associated with encephalitis, herpetic whitlow (pustular lesion on the hand), esophagitis, and pneumonia. HSV-2 is associated with aseptic meningitis and neonatal herpes.

TOP SECRET

ID/CC	A 72-year-old Caucasian male presents with a **painful rash** on the right side of his chest.
HPI	The patient has been taking medication for high blood pressure but is otherwise in excellent health. He also reports **severe burning pain preceding the appearance of the rash.**
PE	VS: low-grade fever (38.1°C). PE: unilateral vesicular eruption **confined to the right T6 dermatome.**
Labs	Tzanck smear of vesicle base reveals large **multinucleated epithelial giant cells.**
Pathogenesis	The causative agent is **varicella-zoster virus** (VZV), a double-stranded DNA virus of the herpesvirus family that causes two distinct pathologies: chickenpox (VARICELLA) and herpes zoster (SHINGLES). Chickenpox is a benign primary infection that is usually seen in children; herpes zoster results from **reactivation of the latent virus** and presents as a **dermatomal, painful vesicular rash.** When branches of the trigeminal nerve are involved, lesions may also appear in the mouth or tongue, around the eye (ZOSTER OPHTHALMICUS), and on the face. The precise mechanism of VZV reactivation is unknown, but it is thought that the virus remains latent in the dorsal root ganglion after a chickenpox infection; the dermatomes from T3 to L3 are most frequently involved.
Epidemiology	Herpes zoster can occur at all ages but primarily affects the elderly. Immunosuppressed patients are also at greater risk of more severe or disseminated infection.
Management	**Analgesics** for pain. **Antivirals** (e.g., acyclovir), especially in zoster ophthalmicus, immune-compromised hosts, and **HIV-positive patients.** Give antibiotics for overlying skin infections; steroids may reduce inflammation and pain.
Complications	Possible ophthalmic problems include conjunctivitis, keratitis, uveitis, and ocular muscle palsies; cerebral angiitis may result in focal neurologic deficits or ataxia. Other complications include postherpetic neuralgia and Ramsay Hunt syndrome. Disseminated disease may develop in immune-compromised patients (particularly lymphoma patients).

INFECTIOUS DISEASE

ID/CC A 40-year-old **cave explorer** complains of **chronic dry cough, malaise, weight loss**, and **night sweats**.

HPI The patient is also a chronic **smoker** but has no history of hemoptysis and has not experienced significant shortness of breath. The patient states that he grew up in the **Ohio River Valley** in the United States.

PE VS: **fever** (38.5°C). PE: scattered rales over both lung fields.

Labs CBC/PBS: anemia; leukopenia. Sputum culture yields *Histoplasma capsulatum*; complement fixation test for histoplasmosis reveals significantly raised titer.

Imaging CXR: bronchopneumonia or multiple nodules are seen in primary form; apical fibronodular changes similar to TB in chronic form. XR, abdomen: calcification in the splenic area (seen in disseminated form).

Pathogenesis The causative agent is *Histoplasma capsulatum*, a sporulating, dimorphic fungus that grows in soil (especially **soil enriched with the fecal material of chickens, starlings, and bats**); infection is acquired via **inhalation of spores** (due to aerosolization of fungus-laden soil). The organism has an affinity for fixed and circulating phagocytic cells of the reticuloendothelial system.

Epidemiology Histoplasmosis is **endemic in the eastern-central United States**; the center of disease activity is within the Ohio and Mississippi river valleys. Although histoplasmosis has long been associated with farming and rural life, epidemic histoplasmosis has been increasingly reported among urban and suburban populations; the common denominator has been the disturbance of soil in and around a starling roost or accumulations of bat droppings.

Management **Most patients** with primary pulmonary disease **do not require therapy**. Severely ill or immune-compromised patients and those with disseminated disease can be effectively treated with **amphotericin B** or **itraconazole**.

Complications **Disseminated histoplasmosis** develops rarely. Clinical disseminated histoplasmosis may present as a systemic illness with multiple-organ-system involvement that includes hepatosplenomegaly, generalized lymphadenopathy, fever, night sweats, anorexia, weight loss, anemia, and leukopenia. Adrenal insufficiency has been noted in 50% of these patients. In immune-compromised patients, progressive disseminated histoplasmosis is an important opportunistic infection. Chronic cavitary histoplasmosis affects middle-aged and elderly men who have severe COPD. Clinically, the disease is similar to cavitary tuberculosis.

CASE 20

ID/CC   A **15-year-old** female complains of **malaise, fatigue**, and loss of appetite for the past week.

HPI   She also complains of mild **fever** and **sore throat**. Her boyfriend recently experienced similar symptoms that lasted approximately 3 weeks.

PE   VS: mild tachycardia; low-grade **fever** (38.2°C). PE: firm, discrete, tender, nonmatted cervical **lymphadenopathy** and **pharyngitis** with marked erythema and a diffuse exudate; **petechiae at junction of hard and soft palate**; no hepatomegaly but **mild soft splenomegaly**.

Labs   CBC: leukocytosis with > 50% lymphocytes and monocytes. [**Fig. 20**] PBS: > 10% **atypical lymphocytes**. Monospot test for **heterophil antibodies positive**; specific EBV antibodies (EA, VLA, EBNA) also positive.

Pathogenesis   The causative agent is **Epstein–Barr virus (EBV)**, a B-lymphotrophic human herpesvirus; it is transmitted primarily by **salivary contact** (as in kissing) and shed intermittently by all seropositive (clinical and subclinical) individuals. Infectious mononucleosis (IM) is defined as the **triad of pharyngitis, fever, and lymphadenopathy combined with heterophil antibodies and atypical lymphocytosis**. A similar disease syndrome may be produced by other infections, such as toxoplasmosis, CMV, and HIV.

Epidemiology   Approximately 50% of the world's population has experienced a primary EBV infection before adolescence. Early infections are usually mild and subclinical, but a second wave of infection occurs at adolescence or

Figure 20

adulthood that accounts for most cases of IM. The peak incidence of IM is 14 to 16 years for girls and 16 to 18 years for boys. EBV is associated with **nasopharyngeal carcinoma, Burkitt's lymphoma,** certain types of **B-cell lymphomas** (especially in immunosuppressed individuals), and hairy leukoplakia in AIDS patients.

Management

Supportive care, adequate bed rest. **Glucocorticoids** may hasten the resolution of pharyngitis and are indicated for airway obstruction, severe thrombocytopenia, CNS involvement, or hemolytic anemia. **Acyclovir, ganciclovir,** and **α-interferon** are potent inhibitors of EBV replication and halt oropharyngeal shedding; however, clinical benefits are minimal. Avoid contact sports for 6 to 8 weeks owing to the risk of splenic rupture. Also avoid antibiotics, particularly ampicillin, as it may cause a skin rash that can be a diagnostic clue to EBV infections.

Complications

Complications include hemolytic anemia, thrombocytopenia, Guillain–Barré syndrome, encephalitis, and splenic rupture with trauma. Airway obstruction may result from pharyngeal adenopathy. There is a strong association with Burkitt's lymphoma and increasing evidence that immunosuppressed individuals and bone-marrow allograft recipients may be predisposed to B-cell lymphoma.

ID/CC

A 76-year-old **male** presents to the ER with **confusion** and a **severe cough.**

HPI

The patient's illness began with the **abrupt onset of headache, muscle aches, and weakness** followed 24 hours later by **high fevers and shaking chills.** He subsequently developed a **nonproductive cough with pleuritic chest pain, dyspnea, nausea, vomiting,** and **diarrhea.** He is a chronic **smoker** and **drinks** heavily.

PE

VS: **high fever** (40.0°C); **bradycardia** (HR 50); tachypnea; normal BP. PE: disoriented; diaphoretic; **crackles bilaterally.**

Labs

CBC: **elevated WBC** (18,000). Lytes: **hyponatremia.** Gram stain of sputum reveals numerous neutrophils but no bacteria; **increased** *Legionella* titers by IFA. Culture on charcoal yeast extract medium positive for *Legionella.*

Imaging

CXR: patchy bronchopneumonia.

Pathogenesis

The causative agent is *Legionella pneumophila,* a gram-negative aerobic bacillus that frequently resides in **environmental water sources;** acquired via **inhalation.** Infection is established in the presence of immunosuppression and/or impaired mucociliary clearance (as in smoking). Person-to-person transmission generally does not occur.

Epidemiology

Older age, smoking, and **depressed cell-mediated immunity** predispose to the development of this infection. The overall mortality rate is approximately 15%.

Management

Erythromycin is the drug of choice. Administer **rifampin in immune-compromised or severely ill patients.** Alternative antibiotics that may be effective include levofloxacin, azithromycin, and clarithromycin.

Complications

Dehydration, extrapulmonary infections, lung abscess, empyema, respiratory failure, pericarditis, endocarditis, myocarditis, shock, DIC, thrombotic thrombocytopenic purpura, peritonitis, renal failure, pyelonephritis, and pancreatitis.

INFECTIOUS DISEASE

ID/CC	A 22-year-old military recruit presents with **altered mental status** following a bout of **high-grade fever**.
HPI	Three days ago the patient had reported that he felt ill and complained of **headache, stiff neck**, a severe cough, a sore throat, chills, and muscle aches.
PE	VS: hypotension (BP 82/40); **tachycardia** (HR 133); **fever** (39.6°C); tachypnea (RR 28). PE: **purpuric lesions** noted over axillae, flanks, wrists, and ankles; no papilledema.
Labs	CBC: **leukopenia**. LP: CSF with low glucose, high protein, and many PMNs. **Gram-negative diplococci** on Gram stain; platelet count and circulating clotting factors decreased; blood culture yields **meningococci**.
Pathogenesis	The causative agent is *Neisseria meningitidis*, a gram-negative diplococcus; spread by droplet infection and disseminated hematogenously from the nasopharynx. Produces the **Waterhouse–Friderichsen syndrome**, characterized by **meningitis, sepsis**, and **adrenal necrosis** (leading to fulminant vasomotor collapse and shock).
Epidemiology	Usually responsible for epidemic cases in the elderly population; however, any age group may be affected. A variable percentage of the population may carry the organism in the nasopharynx.
Management	**Aggressive IV fluid and steroid replacement** is key in vasomotor collapse secondary to adrenal failure. Administer cardiovascular or respiratory support as necessary. **Penicillin is the drug of choice** in meningococcal infection; third-generation cephalosporins (e.g., ceftriaxone) may be given for empiric therapy, and chloramphenicol for β-lactam-allergic patients. Administer **rifampin prophylaxis for all household contacts**. Vaccination is recommended for immunodeficient or asplenic patients, those traveling to endemic areas, and military recruits.
Complications	Fulminant meningococcemia with shock, peripheral gangrene, DIC, acidosis, brain injury (due to meningitis), and long-term adrenal insufficiency.

ID/CC A 58-year-old male develops **pleuritic chest pain, fever,** and **shaking chills.**

HPI He also complains of a cough with **purulent sputum** formation. He is a chronic heavy **smoker with COPD.** He reports having had a **URI 1 week ago** with cough, coryza, and conjunctivitis.

PE VS: **high fever** (39.4°C); tachycardia (HR 117); tachypnea (RR 23); normal BP. PE: mild respiratory distress; **decreased breath sounds, inspiratory rales, dullness to percussion,** and **increased tactile fremitus** over right lower lung field.

Labs CBC: **leukocytosis** (17,500) with **neutrophilia** (84%). Elevated ESR. Lytes: normal. Sputum Gram stain shows **gram-positive diplococci in pairs** and many PMNs; sputum culture confirms *Streptococcus pneumoniae* (positive in only 25% of patients); blood cultures usually negative (positive in only 25% of patients).

Imaging [**Fig. 23A**] CXR: lobar consolidation in the right upper lobe bounded inferiorly by the horizontal fissure. [**Fig. 23B**] CT, chest: a different case in which an air bronchogram (1) is seen in area of consolidation (2).

Pathogenesis *S. pneumoniae* lung infection is a major cause of **lobar pneumonia** and typically affects those who are at the **extremes of age** or those who have an underlying disease. For example, asplenic patients are unable to efficiently clear nonopsonized bacteria from the blood.

Epidemiology Pneumococcal pneumonia usually follows a URI and is more common in patients with chronic cardiopulmonary disease as well as in sickle cell disease and asplenic (or splenectomized) patients, in whom disease is more severe. It is also more common among smokers, renal-failure

INFECTIOUS DISEASE

Figure 23A

Figure 23B

patients, alcoholics, and immune-compromised patients (HIV). There is a higher incidence in late winter and early spring.

Management   Hospitalize if the patient is older than 65 years and has concurrent illnesses, is severely ill, or is homeless. Start empiric antibiotics based on likely pathogen. *Pneumococcus* is the most common cause of community-acquired pneumonia (CAP); **penicillin** is the drug of choice. Ceftriaxone, vancomycin, or fluoroquinolones may be effective for the treatment of penicillin-resistant pneumococcal infections. For atypical pneumonia, *Mycoplasma* and *Chlamydia* are common pathogens; a macrolide is the drug of choice. For CAP requiring hospitalization, also consider *Haemophilus influenzae*, gram-negative rods, and *Legionella* as the cause; give second- or third-generation cephalosporin. For nosocomial pneumonia, consider *Pseudomonas, Staphylococcus aureus, Escherichia coli,* and *Klebsiella* as the cause; give empiric therapy with third-generation cephalosporin and aminoglycoside. Prevent with pneumococcal vaccine for patients who undergo splenectomy as well as those who have malignancies, sickle cell disease, or COPD.

Complications   Atelectasis, bacteremia, meningitis, parapneumonic pleural effusion, lung abscess, pericarditis, and empyema.

ID/CC   A 23-year-old woman complains of the appearance of a **prominent diffuse rash** over the past 2 to 3 days.

HPI   The patient adds that about **1 week** before the rash appeared, she felt tired and had a **low-grade fever**, swollen cheeks and lymph nodes, mild nasal congestion, itchy eyes, and minor **joint aches** in her fingers, wrists, and knees. The rash **started on her face, spread to her trunk, and then spread down her arms and legs**, with each phase lasting about 1 day. She denies any sexual activity and denies the possibility of pregnancy.

PE   VS: normal. PE: **diffuse maculopapular rash; petechial exanthem on soft palate** (FORSCHHEIMER SPOTS) noted along with **patchy erythema** in oropharynx without exudate; mild nasal erythema without exudate; soft, movable **lymphadenopathy** noted in **postauricular** and posterior cervical distribution.

Labs   ELISA demonstrates **rubella-specific IgM and IgG antibodies** (acute rubella shows fourfold or higher increase in IgG titer). CBC: thrombocytopenia. Pregnancy test negative.

Pathogenesis The causative agent is rubella virus, a **togavirus**. Transmission is via droplets shed in respiratory secretions, infecting the respiratory tract and, subsequently, the bloodstream, resulting in the characteristic rash, fever, and lymphadenopathy.

Epidemiology Owing to greater than 95% seroconversion of vaccinated individuals, routine use of the live attenuated vaccine has virtually eliminated epidemic outbreaks of rubella among school-age children; **most cases now occur in young adults**. Although it is often subclinical, rubella is highly contagious, albeit less so than measles; it is transmissible via **respiratory droplets** from 1 week prior to the appearance of the rash to 15 days afterward, with the incubation period ranging from 14 to 21 days (average 18 days). Natural infection leads to lifelong immunity; antibody to rubella crosses the placenta and thereby protects the newborn.

Management There is **no specific therapy** for rubella; the management of acute rubella consists of the **symptomatic relief** of fever (acetaminophen), arthralgias, arthritis, encephalitis, thrombocytopenia, etc. All infants should be **immunized with live attenuated virus vaccine** (the **first dose administered between 12 and 15 months of age** and **another dose given during childhood**). **Pregnant women should not be immunized**, and birth control should be practiced for a minimum of 3 months following vaccine administration. Consider therapeutic abortion if exposure occurs during pregnancy. **No serious side effects** have been reported after the administration of rubella **vaccine to immune-compromised** individuals.

INFECTIOUS DISEASE

continued

Complications Congenital abnormalities, which include early-onset cataracts, glaucoma, microphthalmia, hearing deficits, heart defects, and psychomotor retardation, occur primarily if the fetus is infected during the first trimester. Rarely, patients (adults more commonly than children) develop postinfectious encephalopathy that begins 1 to 6 days after the appearance of the rash.

CASE 25

ID/CC	A 30-year-old male presents to the dermatology outpatient clinic complaining of a **generalized rash** and **hair loss**.
HPI	The skin eruption is nonpruritic. He reports having had **unprotected sexual intercourse** with multiple partners; on directed questioning he notes that he had a **painless ulcer** (CHANCRE) on his penis a few weeks ago.
PE	**Maculopapular skin rash** over entire body, including **palms and soles**; patches of hair loss involving scalp and eyebrows (FOLLICULAR SYPHILIDES); generalized nontender lymphadenopathy; mucous patches (silver-gray erosions with a red periphery) seen on tongue; **condylomata lata** (broad, moist, gray-white lesions) seen in perianal and intertriginous groin area; edges of skin are indurated (ELLIOT'S SIGN).
Labs	Darkfield examination of specimens obtained from condylomata and mucous patches reveals presence of treponemes; RPR positive; **VDRL titers increased** (> 1:32); FTA-ABS test (confirmatory) positive.
Pathogenesis	Causative agent is *Treponema pallidum*. Usually transmitted during sexual activity by direct contact with the mucocutaneous lesions that arise during the primary or secondary stage of syphilis (tertiary syphilis is rarely transmissible); however, vertical transmission from an untreated pregnant woman (maximum risk during 16 to 36 weeks' gestation) may result in congenital syphilis in the fetus.
Epidemiology	In the United States, the incidence of syphilis diminished markedly from the 1940s through the 1970s as a result of the introduction of antibiotics. Since then there have been two epidemics in the U.S.; the first, which occurred in the early 1980s and primarily involved homosexual and bisexual males, subsequently declined due to sexual behavior modification among this group in response to the risk of AIDS. The second epidemic, which occurred during the second half of the 1980s, primarily involved women, adolescents, and heterosexuals who exchanged sex for drugs or money. Approximately **one-half** of those involved in sexual activity with individuals infected with syphilis become infected.
Management	**Benzathine penicillin G** administered intramuscularly; if patient is sensitive to penicillin, erythromycin or doxycycline can be used. **Follow up with VDRL levels.** The CSF should be examined if the VDRL titer does not become negative or does not decrease dramatically in 6 months; if the CSF is abnormal, treat as for neurosyphilis. If relapse develops, patients should also be tested for HIV infection.
Complications	Tertiary syphilis, which includes neurosyphilis, Argyll Robertson pupil abnormalities (afferent pupil defect), tabes dorsalis (destruction of posterior spinal columns), and syphilitic aortitis.

INFECTIOUS DISEASE

ID/CC   A 45-year-old male with a history of **untreated venereal disease** complains of **pain in his legs** and **difficulty walking**, especially in the dark.

HPI   For the past year, the patient has noted sporadic episodes of electric-like "lightning" pain in his legs that last for hours or days. He also complains of persistent numbness and tingling (feeling of "pins and needles") in his feet and has been "stumbling" whenever he turns quickly.

PE   VS: normal. PE: **discrepancy in pupillary size** (ANISOCORIA); involved pupil **reacts poorly to light but normally to accommodation** (ARGYLL ROBERTSON PUPIL); cranial nerves grossly intact; motor exam 5/5 bilaterally throughout; DTRs 2+ and symmetric in upper extremities but **absent at patella and Achilles**; Babinski's absent bilaterally; sensory exam reveals **decreased vibratory and proprioception sense** in feet; **Romberg's sign positive**; patient maintains knees in an extended position; finger-to-nose intact bilaterally (tests cerebellar function).

Labs   CBC/Lytes: normal. PT/PTT and glucose normal; **serum FTA-ABS positive.** LP: **lymphocytic pleocytosis**; protein of 80 mg/dL; normal glucose; **positive FTA-ABS; positive oligoclonal bands** (FTA-ABS test is more sensitive and specific for the detection of treponemal antigens than VDRL).

Pathogenesis   Tabes dorsalis is a form of **neurosyphilis** that is characterized by **chronic progressive demyelination** of the posterior column of the spinal cord, posterior sensory ganglia (dorsal root ganglia), and nerve roots. *Treponema pallidum*, a spirochete, is the causative organism; it usually invades the CNS 3 to 18 months after systemic infection occurs.

Epidemiology   The incidence of latent syphilis is 7.4 per 100,000 in the United States.

Management   Treat with **IV penicillin**. If the patient is allergic to penicillin, he should undergo desensitization and then proceed with penicillin. Follow response to therapy by checking LP repeatedly over 2 years. Expect normalization of CSF VDRL by 1 year; relapse after 2 years of negative CSF is uncommon.

Complications   Complications include **Charcot's joints** (joint damage due to decreased sensation of lower limbs), incontinence secondary to neurogenic bladder, painless ulcers over pressure points, hearing loss, and visual loss due to uveitis, chorioretinitis, or optic neuritis. **Tabes crises** consist of abdominal pain and bladder dysfunction.

ID/CC

A 35-year-old **HIV-positive** male complains of **increasing fatigue, weight loss, fever**, and a **progressively worsening cough** of 6 weeks' duration.

HPI

He also acknowledges having **frequent night sweats**. He has no known contacts with tuberculosis but is known to have had **HIV infection** for 3 years; his last CD4 count was 150.

PE

VS: fever (39.5°C). PE: thin, lethargic; oral thrush; mild cervical lymphadenopathy bilaterally; mild rales audible in bilateral apices.

Labs

Sputum cultures positive for **acid-fast bacilli**; PPD and anergy panel nonreactive (secondary to immunosuppression); cultures eventually grow *Mycobacterium tuberculosis*.

Imaging

[**Fig. 27A**] CXR: primary complex with ill-defined right upper lobe consolidation (1) and right paratracheal adenopathy (2). [**Fig. 27B**] CXR: post-primary tuberculosis with right upper lobe consolidation and central cavitation.

Pathogenesis

The causative agent is *Mycobacterium tuberculosis*; infection is acquired **via inhalation of aerosolized droplets** that reach the lungs. The bacteria are then ingested by macrophages and are killed or persist and multiply. Organisms may disseminate to the lymphatic system and bloodstream until they are walled off by granulomatous inflammation (due to **type IV hypersensitivity reaction**). This process of primary infection is typically asymptomatic. Viable organisms remain dormant for years and may reactivate disease when host defenses are compromised. Some disease states and conditions, such as diabetes mellitus, silicosis, postgastrectomy, and immunosuppression, are associated with an increased risk of reactivation.

Epidemiology

The incidence of tuberculosis continues to increase worldwide. The frequency of atypical presentations also continues to increase, particularly

INFECTIOUS DISEASE

Figure 27A

Figure 27B

continued

in the **elderly**, patients with **HIV** infection, and nursing home residents. HIV infection represents the most important risk factor for tuberculosis today, and the recent increase in the incidence of tuberculosis can be attributed to the HIV epidemic. Multi-drug-resistant strains of *M. tuberculosis* are now seen with increasing frequency.

Management   Immediate respiratory isolation. Start treatment with a **four-drug regimen of INH, rifampin, pyrazinamide**, and **ethambutol**. Directly observed therapy is an option for noncompliant patients. A presumptive diagnosis requires acid-fast bacilli on smear or a positive PPD in patients with CXR findings. A culture is required to confirm the diagnosis and to narrow antimycobacterial coverage. Five- or six-drug regimens should be used for outbreaks of strains resistant to INH and rifampin. Give supplemental **oral pyridoxine**, which prevents neuropathy due to vitamin B_6 deficiency caused by INH. **Serum bilirubin, liver enzymes, BUN**, and **creatinine** should be monitored prior to therapy. **Chemoprophylaxis** with INH or rifampin for 12 months should be given to high-risk individuals, close contacts of patients with INH-resistant tuberculosis, patients with positive tuberculin skin tests (< 35 years of age), and any of the following: known or suspected HIV infection, close contacts of newly diagnosed patients, recent converters, and patients with chronic illness. Immunization with BCG (results in a positive PPD) is widely used in developing countries where the incidence of tuberculosis is high, but is not used in the United States at this time.

Complications   Lobar or segmental collapse or consolidation, pleural effusion, pericardial involvement, tuberculoma formation, meningitis, and miliary tuberculosis.

ID/CC A 24-year-old male complains of **persistent fever** of 2 weeks' duration along with mild **abdominal pain, constipation, a skin rash**, and a sore throat and cough.

HPI He additionally complains of malaise, myalgias, arthralgias, and headaches. He reports having traveled to Mexico recently, where he ate **food** from **street vendors**.

PE VS: **bradycardia** (HR 50); **fever** (38.5°C); normal BP. PE: confluent macular **erythematous rash on trunk** that fades on pressure (ROSE SPOTS); abdomen mildly distended and tender but with no peritoneal signs; mild **hepatosplenomegaly**.

Labs CBC: anemia; **neutropenia**. Widal's test reveals **elevated "O" antigen titer** of 1:320 (> 1:160 is diagnostic); blood and stool cultures positive for *Salmonella typhi*. UA: proteinuria; various casts.

Imaging CXR: normal (may show free subdiaphragmatic air in typhoid intestinal perforation).

Pathogenesis The causative agent is *Salmonella typhi*. Typhoid fever predominantly affects human lymphoid tissue; the incubation period is variable (3 to 60 days) and is inversely proportional to the number of bacilli ingested. Infection classically results in **longitudinal ulcers in the ileum** (along Peyer's patches) and perforation (typically after 3 weeks of the disease), with subsequent peritonitis and variable patterns of GI bleeding leading to hypotension and hypovolemic shock.

Epidemiology Typhoid fever has a worldwide distribution but is predominantly a disease of **developing countries** (due to poor sanitation); it is transmitted through **contaminated food or drink** (starchy foods, shellfish, eggs, and beverages, including milk), through **contact with the feces or urine** of patients or asymptomatic carriers (females with typhoid cholecystitis and patients with *Schistosoma hematobium* urine infections are frequently carriers), and by **houseflies** that may act as mechanical vectors. Typhoid fever is associated with significant morbidity and mortality approaching 15%.

Management The primary antibiotic choices include **ceftriaxone** or **ciprofloxacin**. If the patient is in shock, administer dexamethasone before antibiotics. In the event of treatment failure or perforation, **laparotomy with resection** of the affected segment is indicated. Fluoroquinolones are contraindicated in children and pregnant women. Asymptomatic carriers may require cholecystectomy if they fail antibiotic therapy. Prevention involves hygienic/dietary measures; **typhoid vaccine** is advised for those traveling to endemic areas.

Complications Septic shock, intestinal perforation and bleeding, endocarditis, pneumonia, cholecystitis, and meningitis.

INFECTIOUS DISEASE

ID/CC	A 29-year-old **female** complains of **pain on urination** (DYSURIA).
HPI	Directed questioning reveals that the patient has also experienced increased urinary **frequency** and **urgency**.
PE	VS: normal. PE: mild suprapubic tenderness; no costovertebral angle tenderness.
Labs	UA: **leukocyte esterase and nitrate positive; pyuria** without WBC casts; urine culture reveals > 10^5 CFU/mL; gram-negative bacilli identified as *Escherichia coli*.
Pathogenesis	Most UTIs result from bacteria ascending into the bladder from the urethra. *E. coli* is responsible for most (80%) cases of acute infections in patients without catheters, calculi, or urologic abnormalities. Other gram-negative rods, including *Proteus*, *Klebsiella*, and *Enterobacter*, are responsible for a smaller number of infections. Gram-positive cocci (e.g., *Staphylococcus saprophyticus*) also play a role in producing UTIs in sexually active women. UTIs are generally categorized as catheter-associated (usually nosocomial) or non-catheter-associated infections. UTIs may also be classified as those affecting the lower urinary tract (cystitis, urethritis, prostatitis) and those affecting the upper tract (pyelonephritis). Alkaline urine suggests the presence of a urea-splitting organism (most commonly *Proteus*).
Epidemiology	The incidence of UTIs increases with the onset of sexual activity. They are more **prevalent during pregnancy** because of the decreased ureteral tone/ureteral peristalsis and temporary incompetence of the vesicoureteral valves. Ten to twenty percent of the elderly population and up to 50% of institutionalized elderly persons have bacteriuria.
Management	Begin antibiotic therapy (**fluoroquinolones**) until the organism is cultured; then tailor antibiotics. **TMP-SMX** is **no longer** considered a **first-line** regimen owing to the increasing resistance of *E. coli*. **Predisposing factors** such as **vesicoureteral reflux, obstruction, neurogenic bladder**, or **calculi** should be identified and treated if possible. Recurrent infections should be identified to determine whether the same strain or a different strain is responsible for recurrence; patients with repeated infections or recent hospitalizations may harbor resistant strains. Individuals with recurrent infection (more than three infections per year) benefit from daily long-term administration of TMP-SMX. Recommend that patients urinate following sexual intercourse.
Complications	Treatment commonly results in complete resolution of symptoms. Lower tract infections are of concern because they can produce pain, discomfort, and lost time from work. Permanent renal damage may result with ascending infection and resultant pyelonephritis.

ID/CC	A 19-year-old male on his first postoperative day after splenectomy experiences **marked oliguria** (< 20 cc urine/hr) and complains of **malaise, anorexia, and nausea.**
HPI	He was found in **shock** after having been in a motorcycle accident. An immediate laparotomy was performed after rehydration, and a ruptured spleen with a **large hemoperitoneum** was found.
PE	VS: normal. PE: well hydrated; **no suprapubic mass** palpable (enlargement of bladder in cases of postrenal ARF).
Labs	CBC: anemia; **leukocytosis with left shift. Increased BUN and creatinine (BUN/creatinine ratio 10:20).** Lytes: hyperkalemia; hyperphosphatemia. ABGs: **metabolic acidosis.** UA: proteinuria; **renal tubular cell and granular casts**; urine specific gravity 1.012; urinary osmolality < 350 mOsm/kg; Fe_{Na} > 1%; urine sodium > 20 mEq/L.
Imaging	US, renal: no ureteral dilatation or enlargement of the kidney.
Pathogenesis	Acute renal failure (ARF) may be oliguric (< 30 cc/hr) or nonoliguric and is classically divided into prerenal, intrinsic renal, and postrenal. **Prerenal ARF** is caused by a decrease in effective extracellular volume with decreased renal perfusion; it is associated with prolonged vomiting and diarrhea, acute blood loss (traumatic, GI, or gynecologic bleeding), fluid retention with heart disease (CHF), cirrhosis, drugs (NSAIDs, ACE inhibitors), vascular contraction, diuretics, and fluid sequestration (e.g., from pancreatitis, burns, peritonitis). Labs show muddy brown or hyaline casts, a BUN/creatinine ratio > 20, urine sodium < 10 mEq/L, Fe_{Na} < 1%, urine osmolality > 500 mOsm/kg, and urine specific gravity > 1.018. **Renal** (INTRINSIC) **failure** is caused by prolonged ischemia (the most common cause of ATN, as in this case), nephrotoxins (cisplatin, **contrast media, aminoglycosides**), and diffuse renal cortical necrosis. **Postrenal** causes of ARF include any **obstruction to urine flow** from the kidney to the urethra, such as kidney stones, pelvic surgery, bladder or prostate tumors, retroperitoneal fibrosis, pelvic tumors, and urethral stricture.
Management	Insert a **Foley catheter** and measure postvoid volume to rule out obstruction. If the patient is volume depleted, administer isotonic saline solution and wait for diuresis; if euvolemic, administer furosemide or dopamine. **Correct acidosis and electrolyte abnormalities** (hyperkalemia, hyperphosphatemia). Adjust meds according to creatinine clearance. **Dialysis** is indicated in severe hyperkalemia, pulmonary edema, refractory acidosis, fluid overload, pericarditis, and uremic encephalopathy.
Complications	Complications include encephalopathy, GI bleeding (impaired platelet function), salt and fluid overload, pericarditis, severe hyperkalemia, hypocalcemia, increased anion-gap metabolic acidosis, and anemia. Opportunistic infections, poor wound healing, and muscle wasting occur due to the hypercatabolic state that is related to uremia and infection.

NEPHROLOGY/UROLOGY

ID/CC   A 55-year-old female with gram-negative septicemia becomes lethargic and develops **decreased urine output**.

HPI   The patient was started on **IV gentamicin** 3 days ago. She subsequently developed increasing **confusion**.

PE   VS: low-grade fever (38.7°C); tachycardia (HR 110); tachypnea; hypotension (BP 90/50). PE: **disoriented; pericardial rub; asterixis**.

Labs   Lytes: **elevated potassium and phosphate**. Elevated BUN and creatinine; blood cultures reveal gram-negative bacilli. UA: proteinuria; **brownish pigmented granular casts with renal tubular epithelial casts in sediment**; decreased urinary osmolality (< 300 mOsm/kg); specific gravity 1.012; Fe_{Na} > 1%. ABGs: metabolic acidosis.

Pathogenesis   Acute tubular necrosis (ATN) occurs secondary to an **ischemic or nephrotoxic insult**, causing focal tubular epithelial cell necrosis leading to **preglomerular vasoconstriction, tubular obstruction** by necrotic tubular epithelial cells and formed casts, and **tubular back leak**. Consequently, tubular flow decreases and intratubular pressure increases, yielding a lower GFR and ultimately oliguria. Oliguria results in **salt and water retention, hyperkalemia, uremia**, and a **metabolic acidosis**.

Epidemiology   ATN is the **most frequent cause of acute renal failure**. Risk factors are classified as toxic (**radiographic contrast, antibiotics, heavy metals, organic solvents, hemoglobinuria, myoglobinuria**) or ischemic (**decreased cardiac output, hemorrhage, sepsis**).

Management   **Correct the underlying etiology**; monitor fluid balance; restrict protein intake; discontinue offending drugs; correct electrolytes. If hypovolemia exists without evidence of obstruction, volume should be repleted in order to **maintain adequate cardiac output and renal perfusion**. After patients are euvolemic, start **diuretics** to promote urine flow. Uremic pericarditis, encephalopathy, severe hyperkalemia, and overt volume overload are indications for **peritoneal dialysis** or **hemodialysis**.

Complications   Renal failure in ATN often lasts 10 to 20 days, with **complete return to normal** renal functioning. Complications include fluid retention, hyperkalemia, anemia, infections, and uremia. Often fatal if left untreated.

CASE 32

ID/CC   A 44-year-old male with end-stage renal disease on hemodialysis complains of an **inability to move**.

HPI   The patient states that he **missed his dialysis appointment** 2 days ago. Since then he has experienced **progressive weakness**.

PE   VS: normal. PE: patient is awake, alert, and oriented ×3; lungs clear to auscultation; normal heart rate and rhythm; normal S_1 and S_2; 0/5 muscle strength in lower extremities with negative DTRs (FLACCID PARALYSIS); 1/5 strength in upper extremities; CN II–XII intact.

Labs   Lytes: **elevated potassium (6.8 mEq/L)**. ECG: **prolonged PR interval and QRS duration; peaked T waves**.

Pathogenesis   Intracellular potassium levels are approximately 150 mEq/L, whereas extracellular levels are ordinarily about 4 mEq/L; an intracellular-to-extracellular shift may lead to profound hyperkalemia. Causes include insulin deficiency, acidosis, hyperosmolality, cell lysis, and succinyl-choline therapy. Potassium levels are generally regulated by the kidney, so **derangements in renal function** (end-stage renal disease, aldosterone deficiency, aldosterone resistance) may also lead to alterations in potassium levels.

Management   ECG changes necessitate emergent **calcium gluconate** (minutes), **glucose and insulin** (20 to 30 minutes), **sodium bicarbonate**, and nebulized albuterol (a β_2-adrenergic agonist). Stop all potassium intake. The next phase of treatment involves **potassium removal**, which may be accomplished with diuretics, dialysis, or cation exchange resins (Kayexalate). Potassium-sparing diuretics (e.g., spironolactone, amiloride) should be used cautiously in patients with chronic renal failure.

Complications   Failure to treat hyperkalemia leads to progressive cardiac dysfunction, ultimately leading to ventricular tachycardia, fibrillation, asystole, and death.

NEPHROLOGY/UROLOGY

TOP SECRET

ID/CC	A 52-year-old man with rheumatoid arthritis and "borderline diabetes" presents to the outpatient clinic complaining of **abdominal bloating** and **bilateral ankle swelling** of several months' duration.
HPI	The patient has suffered from severe rheumatoid arthritis for more than a decade and has been using **gold therapy** successfully for nearly 2 years. His blood sugar has been "borderline" for the past year.
PE	VS: normal. PE: in no acute distress; no JVD; skin normal; lungs clear; cardiac exam normal; abdomen nontender and distended, with **positive fluid wave and shifting dullness**; extremities notable for **3+ pitting edema** in bilateral lower extremities to midcalves.
Labs	CBC/Lytes: normal. UA: urine dipstick positive for 3+ protein but otherwise negative; 24-hour urine protein excretion 6.7 g/day (nephrotic range proteinuria > 3.0 g/day). **Low serum albumin** (1.9 g/dL) and serum protein (5.4 g/dL); serum and urine electrophoresis negative; **hyperlipidemia**; renal biopsy shows **thickened glomerular basement membrane** and **"spike and dome" pattern** with silver methenamine staining; immunofluorescence reveals finely **granular deposits of IgG and C3** along capillary loops; subepithelial electron-dense deposits seen on electron microscopy; ANA negative; TFTs normal.
Pathogenesis	The precise pathogenic mechanism of membranous glomerulonephritis is unknown; it is associated with a number of disorders, including hepatitis B, autoimmune diseases (SLE, diabetes mellitus, thyroiditis, multiple connective tissue disorders), and carcinoma, as well as with the use of drugs such as gold, penicillamine, and captopril.
Epidemiology	Membranous glomerulonephritis is the **most common cause of primary nephrotic syndrome in adults.** The male-to-female ratio is 2 to 1. The peak is around the fourth and fifth decades of life (almost always occurring after age 30), and an increased incidence of occult neoplasms of the lung, stomach, and colon has been observed in patients older than 50 years.
Management	**Prednisone** with or without cytotoxic agents for 3 months induces remission in some patients, but its efficacy is controversial.
Complications	Slow but progressive loss of renal function over a period of 3 to 10 years may be observed in 10% of patients. Some patients may also develop secondary renal vein thromboses as a complicating feature.

ID/CC

A 7-year-old boy presents with a 2-month history of **lower extremity edema and progressive abdominal distention**.

HPI

The patient has no significant prior medical history, although he had a "**bad cold**" for several weeks that ended approximately 1 month ago. The parents deny any history of allergies, use of NSAIDs, photophobia, arthralgias, or myalgias.

PE

VS: normal. PE: in no acute distress; skin normal; no JVD; thyroid normal; lungs clear; cardiopulmonary exam normal; abdomen distended, with shifting dullness and palpable fluid thrill (due to **ascites**); extremities notable for **2+ pedal** and **ankle edema** bilaterally; normal skin exam.

Labs

CBC/Lytes: normal. Creatinine normal. UA: urine dipstick notable for 3+ proteinuria. **Serum albumin decreased**; serum protein decreased; **hypertriglyceridemia**; 24-hour urine protein 9.7 g/day (nephrotic-range proteinuria ≥ 3.0 g/day); serum and urine electrophoreses negative; ANA negative; following renal biopsy, light microscopy unremarkable; immunofluorescence negative for immunoglobulins; EM reveals "**fusion**" **of epithelial foot processes**.

Imaging

US, abdomen: excess peritoneal fluid (ASCITES).

Pathogenesis

The precise etiology of minimal-change disease remains unknown. It is associated with **recent viral URIs**, immunizations, hypersensitivity reactions to drugs (e.g., NSAIDs), or allergic reactions (e.g., bee stings) and may also occur as a paraneoplastic manifestation of Hodgkin's disease.

Epidemiology

Minimal-change disease is the **most common cause of nephrotic syndrome in children** but is occasionally seen in adults.

Management

Prednisone induces remission in 50% of adults and in 90% of children, but > 50% of patients relapse. Add cyclophosphamide or chlorambucil for relapsed disease. Diuretics are used to decrease severe edema. Although patients with minimal-change disease rarely progress to renal failure, they often develop complications requiring monitoring.

Complications

Patients have demonstrated increased susceptibility to bacterial infections (gram-positive organisms), spontaneous bacterial peritonitis, thromboembolic events, severe hyperlipidemia, and protein malnutrition.

NEPHROLOGY/UROLOGY

ID/CC   A 73-year-old man with adult-onset **diabetes mellitus**, hypertension, and rheumatoid arthritis presents with a decline in **mental status** and **decreased urinary output.**

HPI   The patient has been diabetic for nearly 30 years, with poorly controlled blood sugars despite insulin and oral agents; he has had **ocular disease** and **renal insufficiency** for > 5 years. He currently takes ACE inhibitors, a thiazide diuretic, and calcium channel blockers for hypertension and takes **NSAIDs** for persistent rheumatoid arthritis. He denies any asthma.

PE   VS: no fever (37.1°C); tachycardia (HR 119); tachypnea (RR 28); hypertension (BP 140/84). PE: disoriented; lethargic, moderately responsive, and in mild distress.

Labs   CBC: normal. Lytes: **hyperkalemia; hyperchloremia. Elevated BUN and creatinine.** ABGs: **non-anion-gap metabolic acidosis.** UA: **acidic urine** (pH < 5.5); **urinary anion gap positive**; proximal H^+ secretion normal.

Pathogenesis   Renal tubular acidosis (RTA) results from deficient H^+ secretion in the distal tubule (**type I**), defective bicarbonate reabsorption in the proximal tubule (**type II**), and defective secretion of both potassium and H^+ in the distal nephron (**type IV**). Type IV is due to a generalized distal nephron dysfunction attributable to either insufficient aldosterone production or intrinsic renal disease, causing **aldosterone resistance**; the resulting hyperkalemia decreases proximal tubule ammonia production and reduces H^+ secretion, leading to inadequate excretion of the acid load. These patients produce acidic urine despite reduced H^+ secretion because of inadequate ammonia to buffer the protons in the distal tubule. RTA is diagnosed by laboratory evidence of primary metabolic acidosis, a normal serum anion gap (< 12), a zero or positive urine anion gap, and exclusion of the presence of diarrhea, calcium chloride, or other acids.

Epidemiology   Whereas types I and II RTA are rare, **type IV RTA is a common cause of normal anion-gap metabolic acidosis.** It is seen most commonly in patients with **renal insufficiency** and chronic medical illnesses such as **diabetes mellitus** (with nephropathy), **tubular interstitial renal disease, hypertension**, and AIDS. Drugs such as **NSAIDs, ACE inhibitors, and heparin** can also produce or contribute to type IV RTA.

Management   **Restrict dietary potassium; discontinue aldosterone antagonists** (NSAIDs, ACE inhibitors, heparin). Mineralocorticoid replacement with **fludrocortisone** usually improves hyperkalemia and acidosis but may worsen hypertension; patients with tubular resistance require higher doses, while hypertension and CHF are relative contraindications. **Loop**

continued

diuretics, sodium bicarbonate, and exchange resins can also be used. Acidosis generally improves as the hyperkalemic contribution to decreased ammonia production is corrected.

Complications   Complications of type IV RTA are those of metabolic acidosis and hyperkalemia, including confusion, weakness, paresthesias, paralysis, arrhythmias, and even cardiac arrest when severe.

NEPHROLOGY/UROLOGY

ID/CC   A 28-year-old white **female** presents to the clinic for a routine physical exam.

HPI   On questioning, she notes that she has been urinating more frequently than normal and does not feel as strong as she once did (**polyuria** and **muscle weakness** secondary to hypokalemia caused by hyperaldosteronism).

PE   VS: hypertension (BP 190/100). PE: thin and well developed; **loud, high-pitched, epigastric bruit bilaterally.**

Labs   ABGs: **metabolic alkalosis.** Lytes: hypokalemia (3.0 mEq/L). Captopril test reveals exaggerated plasma renin activity.

Imaging   US, renal artery (duplex): bilateral renal artery stenosis > 50%. [**Fig. 36A**] Angio, renal: a different case showing "**string of beads**" (alternating thick fibromuscular ridges and thin vessel wall) appearance of the right renal artery.

Pathogenesis   Fibromuscular dysplasia is a **disease of small and medium-sized arteries** that is characterized most commonly by **medial hyperplasia with or without elastic membrane fibrosis** (MEDIAL DYSPLASIA). One may also observe periadventitial or intimal dysplasia. The stenosis thus produced

Figure 36A

continued

results in decreased perfusion to the kidney, with subsequent activation of the renin-angiotensin-aldosterone axis. This hormonal activation results in hypertension (action of angiotensin II and volume expansion due to aldosterone) and electrolyte abnormalities secondary to hyperaldosteronism (hypernatremia, hypokalemia, and metabolic alkalosis). Polyuria may result from severe hypokalemia. The right renal artery is involved more frequently than the left.

Epidemiology

This disorder most commonly arises in **females** and **frequently affects the renal and carotid arteries**. It may, however, involve peripheral vasculature, producing symptoms similar to peripheral vascular disease. Rare in blacks.

Management

Percutaneous transluminal angioplasty (cures > 50% of patients); medical management of hypertension (ACE inhibitors).

Complications

Renal scarring secondary to ischemia.

Figure 36B Shrunken kidney with a granular capsule adjacent to aorta with atherosclerosis.

NEPHROLOGY/UROLOGY

ID/CC A 50-year-old woman presents after suffering a **tonic-clonic seizure.**

HPI She also complains of weakness in the right arm and leg and has been experiencing a severe **headache, projectile vomiting,** and **blurring of vision.** She has traveled to **Mexico** within the last 5 years.

PE VS: normal. PE: **papilledema**; motor weakness with increased tone noted in right arm and leg; DTRs exaggerated on right side; plantar response on right side is extensor; multiple nontender subcutaneous nodules noted over abdomen, arms, and neck.

Labs CBC: eosinophilia. **Serum serology for cysticercosis positive.** LP (performed once elevated ICP is lowered): mononuclear cell-predominant pleocytosis; elevated proteins; low glucose.

Imaging MR/CT, head: **multiple ring-enhancing lesions** involving the left cortex surrounded by considerable edema. XR, arm: multiple small soft tissue calcifications known as "puffed rice" lesions.

Pathogenesis The causative agent of cysticercosis is *Taenia solium.* **Intestinal infection** occurs through the **ingestion of undercooked pork containing cysticerci.** Ingestion of *T. solium* eggs may also occur through consumption of **food contaminated** by egg-containing feces or by **autoinfection** involving hand-to-mouth fecal carriage. Clinical presentation depends on the organ compromised by the cysticerci; the most serious forms of cysticercosis are those with **ocular, cardiac,** and **neurologic** involvement.

Epidemiology Most infections are encountered in **developing countries,** where intestinal *T. solium* infections occur frequently. In endemic regions, cysticercosis is the most common cause of seizure disorders.

Management **Praziquantel** and **albendazole** are the mainstays of therapy. Give **corticosteroids** to limit inflammatory reactions to dying cysticerci; these reactions render ocular and spinal cysticercosis untreatable. CT scans should be repeated 3 to 6 months after therapy to evaluate cyst viability, and therapy should be repeated if viable cysts remain.

Complications Seizures, hydrocephalus, and chronic meningitis.

CASE 38

ID/CC A 32-year-old male is brought to the ER with **headache**, nausea, vomiting, and **fever**.

HPI The patient is a former **IV drug user** who also complains of cough and shortness of breath. His next-door neighbor raises **pigeons** as a hobby.

PE VS: **low-grade fever** (38.5°C); tachycardia (HR 146); hypotension (BP 80/55). PE: **altered sensorium; mild nuchal rigidity; papilledema**; oral thrush.

Labs CBC: anemia; lymphopenia; decreased CD4+ T-cell count. LP: CSF with **lymphocytic pleocytosis**, increased protein, and decreased glucose. **India ink** preparation demonstrates round, yeastlike cells; **latex agglutination test for cryptococcal antigen positive**; HIV ELISA positive.

Imaging CXR: lobar disease, pleural effusion, and hilar adenopathy. MR, brain: cerebral atrophy; no communicating hydrocephalus; **scattered focal lesions**.

Pathogenesis The causative agent is *Cryptococcus neoformans*. The **most common opportunistic systemic fungal infection in patients with AIDS**, cryptococcosis is acquired via the respiratory route and disseminated hematogenously to the CNS. It most commonly affects the **meninges**.

Epidemiology In the United States, half of all cases of cryptococcosis are found in **AIDS patients**; of those patients who are not HIV positive, most are **immunosuppressed**. **Pigeon droppings** and eucalyptus trees are considered significant environmental reservoirs.

Management IV amphotericin B with **flucytosine; fluconazole** for maintenance therapy. Begin fluconazole after the CD4+ count drops below 100 cells/μL for candidal and cryptococcal prophylaxis.

Complications With advancing illness, brainstem compression, coma, and death may occur rapidly. Pulmonary cryptococcosis may manifest as chest pain and cough; skin and osteolytic bone lesions may occur. Rarely, hepatitis, endophthalmitis, pericarditis, and endocarditis may occur. Acute renal failure may occur with amphotericin B.

NEUROLOGY

ID/CC

A 36-year-old man presents to the ER complaining of sudden-onset **pain and swelling in his left knee** of 3 hours' duration.

HPI

The patient is a basketball player who reports having had **repeated arthroscopic procedures** on both knees. In addition to his sudden pain, he notes associated **fever and chills**. No other joint involvement was noted, and he denies any prior heart valve disease or intravenous drug use.

PE

VS: fever (39.4°C). PE: back, hip, and ankle exams normal; left knee shows significant **induration, erythema, warmth, and marked tenderness to light palpation**; active range of motion limited by pain; passive range of motion intact; drawer tests negative.

Labs

CBC: **marked leukocytosis** (> 100,000 with > 90% PMNs). Synovial fluid analysis shows **pleocytosis** (> 100,000 with > 90% PMNs) and **low glucose**; Gram stain positive for gram-positive cocci in clusters; culture reveals *Staphylococcus aureus*.

Imaging

XR, knee: normal (normal early, but may manifest demineralization within a few days; complicating features such as osteomyelitis or periostitis may be seen as bony erosions or joint space narrowing within 2 weeks).

Pathogenesis

Septic arthritis is characterized by **acute bacterial infection of a joint** accompanied by a systemic reaction with fever and chills, diagnostic joint fluid findings, evidence of concurrent infection, and response to antibiotics. Etiologically, it is classified as either **gonococcal** (causative agent *Neisseria gonorrhoeae*) or **nongonococcal** (most common causative agent *S. aureus*). Bacteria enter the affected joint via the **bloodstream**, having spread from a **neighboring site of infection** (e.g., bone or soft tissue), or by **direct inoculation**. Gonococcal arthritis, which accounts for up to half of all cases, is distinguished by prodromal migratory polyarthralgias, tenosynovitis, purulent monoarthritis, and a characteristic maculopapular or vesicular rash. Patients may or may not have accompanying GU complaints. Nongonococcal acute bacterial arthritis presents with sudden-onset monoarticular arthritis in weight-bearing joints with large joint effusions and occurs almost exclusively in individuals with known predisposing factors. Infections involving *S. aureus* usually arise after **surgery, penetrating injury**, or **other predisposing factors**.

Epidemiology

Predisposing factors include **damaged joints** (osteoarthritis, rheumatoid arthritis, trauma, repeated procedures or surgeries), **persistent septicemia** (intravenous drug users, endocarditis), **immunosuppression** (malignancy, HIV, end-stage renal disease), and **prosthetic joints** (loss of normal local host defenses).

continued

Management

Administration of **IV penicillinase-resistant β-lactam antibiotics** in combination with third-generation cephalosporin (e.g., cefotaxime or ceftriaxone) provides coverage for most infections. Local measures include hot compresses, joint immobilization (splint/traction), rest, and elevation. The drug of choice for gonococcal arthritis (based on joint aspirate Gram stain) is IV ceftriaxone. Patients with a high suspicion for gonococcal arthritis should be admitted to the hospital immediately to confirm the diagnosis and rule out endocarditis. Gonococcal arthritis responds promptly to antibiotic therapy within 24 to 48 hours, leading to complete recovery in nearly all cases. Nongonococcal arthritis also responds rapidly to antibiotic therapy in the absence of severe underlying disease. Patients are switched to oral cephalosporins or ciprofloxacin following clinical improvement for 24 to 48 hours to finish a 7-day treatment course. **Local aspiration** may be required with persistent reaccumulation of effusions. **Surgical drainage** is indicated with hip involvement (poor access by aspiration) or when medical therapy fails after 2 to 4 days. Early active-motion exercises may hasten recovery.

Complications

Delayed or inadequate treatment may result in permanent articular destruction and bony ankylosis.

Figure 39A Edema and erythema of the left ankle.

Figure 39B Unilateral swelling and erythema of the knee.

ID/CC	A 47-year-old male complains of **severe shortness of breath**.
HPI	The patient was admitted 2 days ago for acute pancreatitis.
PE	VS: **fever** (38.5°C); **tachycardia** (HR 112); **tachypnea** (RR 30–36); hypotension. PE: altered mental status; **central cyanosis**; warm, moist skin; accessory muscles (sternocleidomastoid and scalenes) used for respiration with intercostal retractions (respiratory distress); **bilateral inspiratory rales** and coarse breath sounds.
Labs	CBC: leukocytosis. ABGs: **severe hypoxemia** (< 70 mmHg) **refractory to increased FIo$_2$; ratio of Pao$_2$ to FIo$_2$ less than 200:1.** Swan–Ganz catheter reveals **pulmonary capillary wedge pressure < 18 mmHg** (noncardiogenic pulmonary edema); elevated amylase and lipase.
Imaging	[Fig. 40] CXR: **diffuse bilateral alveolar and interstitial infiltrates** with normal heart size. Echo: **normal LV function**.
Pathogenesis	Adult respiratory distress syndrome (ARDS) represents a common pathway for many pathologic processes (sepsis, shock, massive trauma, DIC, pneumonia, burns, oxygen toxicity, emboli) that lead to **increased capillary permeability** and consequent **extravasation of intraluminal contents into the interstitium and eventually the alveoli**, leading to

Figure 40

continued

pulmonary edema and atelectasis. The presence of vascular contents, especially fibrinogen, within the alveoli leads to **deranged surfactant production and fibrinolysis**, allowing for the formation of **hyaline membranes**. Eventually, this leads to **decreased lung compliance**, requiring greater inspiratory pressures, which translates into increased work of breathing.

Management

Endotracheal intubation and **mechanical ventilation** with positive end-expiratory pressure (PEEP) and **supplemental oxygen; IV fluids** for hypotension; DVT prophylaxis (SC heparin). **Nutritional supplementation** is needed because patients have an increased basal metabolism. **Antibiotics** for treatment of underlying sepsis.

Complications

Patients often suffer from multisystem organ failure, DIC, sepsis, or shock. ARDS ultimately leads to death in **50% to 60% of cases**. Patients who do survive generally recover 90% of their previous pulmonary function within the first year, but they may suffer oxygen toxicity secondary to long-term administration of > 50% FIo_2. Complications of PEEP include spontaneous pneumothorax and reduced cardiac output.

PULMONARY

ID/CC A 69-year-old white male who is a retired **shipyard worker** complains of a feeling of **breathlessness, initially on exertion and now even at rest.**

HPI The patient states that he worked for over **30 years in construction,** focusing primarily on the restoration of **old buildings.** He states that he has had a dry cough for years along with worsening fatigue, anorexia, and weight loss. He denies any history of smoking.

PE VS: no fever; tachycardia (HR 115); tachypnea (RR 30); normal BP. PE: clubbing; **dry end inspiratory fine bibasilar crackles;** loud P_2, parasternal heave (RVH) and JVD (secondary to pulmonary hypertension).

Labs Sputum examination reveals **asbestos bodies.** PFTs: **reduced total lung capacity, vital capacity, residual volume, and DL_{CO};** normal FEV_1/FVC.

Imaging CXR: ground-glass appearance and small linear opacities (septal lines) most pronounced at bases. [**Fig. 41A**] CXR: large, irregular, calcified **pleural plaques** are seen bilaterally. [**Fig. 41B**] CT, chest: a different case demonstrates calcified pleural plaques, especially over the right hemidiaphragm.

Pathogenesis Asbestosis is a **diffuse interstitial fibrosing disease** that follows prolonged inhalation of any asbestiform fiber. Alveolar macrophages phagocytose these fibers and undergo membrane damage. Lysosomal enzymes are subsequently liberated, damaging the parenchyma of the lung, which heals by **scarring** and **fibrosis** and produces diffuse interstitial fibrosis. With advanced disease, the acinar units are eventually obliterated, forming a "**honeycombed lung.**" Asbestos-related pleural disease is the most common manifestation of chronic exposure to asbestos and is completely benign.

Figure 41A

Figure 41B

continued

Epidemiology

Asbestosis occurs primarily in individuals who have at least 10 years of moderate to severe **exposure to asbestos**, usually in the workplace (miners, shipyard workers, boilermakers, mill workers), and there is a 20- to 30-year **latency period**. Asbestos exposure is also associated with an increased risk of **malignant mesothelioma** (both pleural and peritoneal) and **lung cancer** (increased risk in chronic smokers).

Management

There is no definitive treatment for asbestosis or mesothelioma; thus, pulmonary physiotherapy, **elimination of exposure**, and **smoking cessation** are crucial.

Complications

Among patients with a history of cigarette smoking, the incidence of both **squamous cell** and **adenocarcinoma of the lung** is elevated approximately **55-fold**. Death usually occurs with onset of asbestosis-related symptoms within 12 to 24 months and may be earlier if Caplan's syndrome, pulmonary hypertension, or cor pulmonale develops.

PULMONARY

TOP SECRET

ID/CC

A 30-year-old man presents to the emergency room with an acute attack of **shortness of breath, coughing, and wheezing.**

HPI

The patient states that the attack occurred several hours after he played with a neighbor's **cat.** Review of systems is positive for **allergic rhinitis, postnasal drip, atopic dermatitis,** and **GERD.**

PE

VS: no fever; **tachycardia** (HR 130); **tachypnea** (RR 40); **pulsus paradoxus.** PE: **confused** and **diaphoretic; uses accessory muscles** of respiration; cyanosis; lungs hyperresonant to percussion; inspiratory and expiratory **diffuse wheezing** bilaterally; increased E:I ratio.

Labs

CBC: **eosinophilia.** ABGs: primary **respiratory alkalosis** with **reduced Po_2 and Pco_2** (elevated Pco_2 indicates respiratory failure); **peak flows decreased.** PFTs: **low FEV_1/FVC** with > 15% improvement of FEV_1 following administration of β_2-agonist; sputum analysis reveals **Curschmann's spirals** (mucus that forms casts in small airways) and **Charcot–Leyden crystals** (eosinophil breakdown products); elevated serum IgE.

Imaging

CXR: hyperinflation, flattened diaphragms (secondary to air trapping and increased residual volume).

Pathogenesis

Bronchial asthma is characterized by airway constriction secondary to reversible, episodic contractions of airway smooth muscle due to **hyper-reactivity,** hypersecretion of **tenacious mucus,** and **mucosal edema** (due to inflammation). It may occur as a response to an allergen **(type I hypersensitivity reaction)** or may be **intrinsic.** Acute attacks may be precipitated by cold air or pollution, smoking, airway infections, emotional stress, and exercise.

Epidemiology

Afflicts 4% to 5% of the population. Children often have the **atopic** form (which may remit in the second decade), whereas intrinsic and occupational asthma arises more commonly in adults.

Management

Manage acute exacerbations with O_2, appropriate respiratory support (including mechanical ventilation if necessary), nebulized β-agonists (e.g., albuterol) and ipratropium, systemic steroids, and antibiotics if indicated in cases with underlying infection. Prophylactic therapy may include **inhaled corticosteroids** (beclomethasone), cromolyn sodium (particularly in children with extrinsic asthma), **leukotriene inhibitors,** and, in severe cases, oral steroids.

Complications

Asthma may lead to **unremitting bronchospasm** (status asthmaticus), **respiratory failure,** respiratory arrest, and death. Patients are also prone to develop recurrent respiratory infections and pneumothorax.

ID/CC

A 56-year-old male presents with **shortness of breath** and a **chronic cough** productive of **copious mucoid sputum**.

HPI

Over the **past 3 years**, his symptoms have occurred for at least 3 months out of every year. He also reports a 40-pack-year **smoking history**.

PE

VS: **tachypnea** (RR 25). PE: **blue lips** (CENTRAL CYANOSIS); plethora; bilateral rhonchi and wheezes.

Labs

CBC: hematocrit increased. ABGs: **hypoxia** and **hypercapnia**. ECG: presence of P-pulmonale and poor progression of R wave in chest leads. PFTs: **obstructive** pattern of increased residual volume and decreased FEV_1/FVC.

Imaging

CXR, PA: presence of increased basilar bronchovascular markings and thickened bronchial walls.

Pathogenesis

The pathologic hallmark of chronic bronchitis is **enlargement of the mucous glands** in the major bronchi. The diameter of the mucous glands relative to the thickness of the bronchial wall (the Reid index) is typically increased from values of 0.26 to 0.44 in healthy persons to > 0.50 in patients with chronic bronchitis. **Smoking** and **occupational exposure** to harmful substances are the principal etiologic factors.

Epidemiology

Seen primarily in smokers.

Management

Smoking cessation and long-term administration of **supplemental oxygen** are the two most important interventions. **Bronchodilators, antibiotics, and corticosteroids** may be used in acute exacerbations.

Complications

Cor pulmonale.

TOP SECRET

CASE 44

ID/CC   A 60-year-old male complains of progressive **shortness of breath on exertion** and a **nonproductive cough**.

HPI   He has a 60-pack-year **smoking history**.

PE   VS: no fever; **tachypnea** (RR 24). PE: moderate **respiratory distress**; **pursed lips**; using **accessory muscles** of respiration; **barrel-shaped chest**; **hyperresonant percussion** note; distant breath sounds; scattered rhonchi heard bilaterally on auscultation; heart sounds distant.

Labs   ABGs: mild hypoxia with hypocapnia. PFTs: **decreased FEV_1/FVC ratio**; decreased DL_{CO}; increased TLC, FRC, and RV.

Imaging   [**Fig. 44A**] CXR, PA: hypertranslucent lung fields with large bullae (1); flattening of the diaphragm (2) and elongated tubular heart shadow. [**Fig. 44B**] CT, chest: multiple large bullae (1). [**Fig. 44C**] CT, chest: innumerable smaller bullae.

Pathogenesis   Emphysema is abnormal permanent **enlargement of air spaces distal to the terminal bronchiole** accompanied by the **destruction of the alveolar**

Figure 44A

Figure 44B

Figure 44C

continued

walls. It may involve the acinus and the lobule uniformly (panacinar) or may primarily involve the respiratory bronchioles (centriacinar). Panacinar emphysema is common in patients with α_1-antitrypsin deficiency. Typically, the lower lobes show more involvement than the upper lobes. **Centriacinar** emphysema is commonly found in cigarette smokers and is rare in nonsmokers. It is usually more extensive and severe in the upper lobes. Emphysema leads to a **reduction in elastic recoil** in the lung that leads to narrowing of the airways with a subsequent decrease in expiratory flow rates (airway obstruction).

Epidemiology   Chronic airway obstruction (CAO) is a leading cause of death in the United States and is second only to CAD as a Social Security-compensated disability. From **80% to 90% of cases of CAO can be attributed to cigarette smoking**; a small percentage is attributable to α_1-antitrypsin deficiency. The risk of death from emphysema or chronic bronchitis is 30 times greater for heavy smokers (> 25 cigarettes/day) than for nonsmokers.

Management   Smoking cessation and long-term administration of **supplemental oxygen** are the two most important interventions. **Bronchodilators** are commonly used; **antibiotics** in acute exacerbations; **corticosteroids** in resistant cases. Influenza and pneumococcal vaccines are recommended. Lung volume reduction surgery and lung transplantation are promising treatments. Surgical excision of bullae may be necessary to provide relief.

Complications   Chronic hypoxemia causes **secondary erythrocytosis** and contributes to exercise limitation, pulmonary hypertension, right heart failure, spontaneous pneumothorax from rupturing of blebs and bullae, and impaired neuropsychiatric function.

CASE 45

ID/CC   A **28-year-old man** presents to the outpatient clinic with complaints of **acute-onset** right-sided **chest pain** and **shortness of breath** that started yesterday afternoon.

HPI   The pain and dyspnea are localized to the right side, are unrelated to position or activity, and actually started while the patient was resting. His symptoms have been stable over the past day, and he has had no progressive difficulty breathing. He has no prior medical or family history but reports that he has **smoked** approximately one pack of cigarettes per day for 7 years.

PE   VS: mild tachycardia. PE: **tall and thin**; in mild distress; no JVD or lymphadenopathy; **diminished breath sounds, decreased tactile fremitus**, and **hyperresonance** in right lung fields; no mediastinal or tracheal shift or cyanosis noted; cardiac exam normal.

Labs   ABGs: **hypoxemia**, acute respiratory alkalosis. ECG: unremarkable.

Imaging [**Fig. 45A**] and [**Fig. 45B**] CXR: the diagnostic **visceral pleural line** is seen on the right side; peripheral to this, the area is seen to be **hyperlucent**, as the lung has retracted.

Figure 45A

Figure 45B

continued

Pathogenesis

Pneumothorax represents an accumulation of air in the pleural space and is classified as spontaneous or traumatic. It is believed to occur as a result of the **rupture of subpleural apical blebs** in response to **high negative intrapleural pressure**. Spontaneous pneumothorax is most commonly primary (without an underlying cause) but may be secondary to pre-existing pulmonary disease (COPD, asthma, cystic fibrosis, TB) and occurs predominantly in smokers. Traumatic pneumothorax results from penetrating or nonpenetrating trauma, often from iatrogenic causes (e.g., thoracocentesis, pleural biopsy, positive-pressure mechanical ventilation).

Epidemiology

Pneumothorax typically affects **tall, thin men** in their **third and fourth decades**. Prior history of *Pneumocystis carinii* pneumonia and use of aerosolized pentamidine are particularly notable risk factors for pneumothorax.

Management

Patients with a small new pneumothorax should be hospitalized, placed on bed rest, given oxygen, and monitored with serial chest x-rays. Small pneumothoraces often resolve spontaneously but may progress unpredictably to tension pneumothorax, which is treated by immediate insertion of a large-bore needle in the affected side, followed by **tube thoracostomy**. Patients with tension or secondary pneumothorax, those with severe symptoms, or those with a large pneumothorax should undergo **chest tube placement** (tube thoracostomy). The chest tube is placed to water-seal suction until the lung begins to expand. Air leaks, recurrence, and pulmonary edema may occur. Patients should be advised to **stop smoking**, as the risk of recurrence is 50% in patients who smoke. High altitudes, flying in unpressurized aircraft, and scuba diving should also be avoided. Thoracoscopy or open thoracotomy with stapling or laser pleurodesis is indicated with recurrent spontaneous pneumothorax, any bilateral pneumothorax, or failure of tube thoracostomy. Scarification by abrasion of the pleural surface may produce pleural symphysis.

Complications

Approximately 30% of patients with spontaneous pneumothorax develop recurrent episodes regardless of initial therapy (observation versus tube thoracostomy). Recurrence is uncommon following surgical interventions. Spontaneous pneumothorax may be complicated by **pneumomediastinum or subcutaneous emphysema**; a secondary ruptured esophagus or bronchus should be ruled out. Tension pneumothorax may rarely be complicated by acute respiratory failure, cardiopulmonary arrest, or death.

PULMONARY

ID/CC   A 40-year-old African-American female complains of progressive **dyspnea on exertion, cough, chest discomfort, weight loss**, and loss of appetite.

HPI   The patient also complains of a purplish rash over her face. Her symptoms have progressed over the past year. She is a **nonsmoker**.

PE   VS: low-grade fever (38.2°C); tachypnea. PE: mild **respiratory distress; bluish-purple, swollen lesions** on nose, cheeks, and earlobes (LUPUS PERNIO); clubbing; bilateral fine inspiratory crackles.

Labs   CBC: lymphopenia. ESR elevated; **hypercalcemia**; hyperglobulinemia; serum **ACE levels elevated**. UA: 24-hour urine calcium elevated. Skin and transbronchial lung biopsies reveal **noncaseating granulomas**; staining and cultures negative for organisms. PFTs: reduced DL_{CO}; reduced FEV_1 and FVC; FEV_1/FVC ratio normal (**restrictive pattern of disease**); Kveim–Siltzbach test (antigen from human sarcoid tissue injected intradermally) positive.

Imaging   [Fig. 46A] CXR: **bilateral hilar lymphadenopathy**. [Fig. 46B] Later stage of lymphadenopathy (1) and reticulonodular densities. HRCT: presence of lymphadenopathy and pulmonary fibrosis confirmed. Nuc: gallium-67 lung scan positive (demonstrates diffuse uptake).

Pathogenesis   The etiology of sarcoidosis is unknown. Accumulation of T cells, macrophages, and noncaseating granulomas in affected organs are seen, probably secondary to an exaggerated immune response to self-antigens or persistent foreign antigens. Organs most commonly affected are the **lungs, skin, eye, and lymph nodes**.

Epidemiology   Sarcoidosis occurs worldwide but is 10 times more prevalent and severe among **African Americans** than among whites. Individuals 20 to 40 years

Figure 46A

Figure 46B

continued

old are most often affected, with a slightly higher prevalence found among females. It is more common in **temperate climates** than in tropical zones and has a higher incidence among **nonsmokers**.

Management

Most patients are asymptomatic or undergo spontaneous remission within 2 years. Use **corticosteroids** for symptomatic pulmonary involvement, systemic symptoms, hypercalcemia, or involvement of extrapulmonary tissues that leads to organ dysfunction, iritis, and CNS and cardiac involvement. **Immunosuppressants** (e.g., methotrexate, azathioprine) may be effective. Regular clinical evaluation is required.

Complications

Neurologic (peripheral neuropathy, cranial nerve palsies, papilledema, meningitis, epilepsy, cerebellar ataxia), cardiac (arrhythmias, CHF, cardiomyopathy), and ocular (anterior or posterior uveitis) manifestations may occur. Hypopituitarism, arthritis, cor pulmonale, and nephrocalcinosis occur as well.

PULMONARY

ID/CC

A 52-year-old man presents with increasing **shortness of breath on exertion**.

HPI

The patient's medical history includes no cardiac or pulmonary disease. He has been working in the **stone-cutting** industry for more than 25 years. His dyspnea on exertion has progressed over many years, and he denies any smoking, alcohol use, or illicit drug use. His family history is unremarkable.

PE

VS: normal. PE: well developed and in no acute distress; no JVD, carotid bruits, or lymphadenopathy; **fine inspiratory crackles at the bases of lungs bilaterally**; cardiac exam normal with no extra heart sounds or murmurs; extremities notable only for **digital clubbing**; no cyanosis or edema.

Labs

PFTs: mild obstructive and restrictive disease and decreased DL_{CO}.

Imaging

CXR: diffuse ground-glass, nodular infiltrates with small, rounded opacities (silicotic nodules) throughout the lung; **peripheral calcifications in hilar lymph nodes** ("EGGSHELL CALCIFICATIONS") may be noted. CT, chest: multiple small nodules.

Pathogenesis

Silicosis represents a diffuse fibrotic reaction of the lungs to inhalation of free crystalline silica particles that are ingested by alveolar macrophages, which rupture and subsequently release cytotoxic enzymes. The silica is reingested by other macrophages, continuing a cycle of cytotoxic enzyme release and progressive local fibrotic reactions, ultimately producing acellular fibrous nodules characteristic of the clinical disease. Long-term exposure over 15 to 20 years results in fibrosis that is sufficient to produce characteristic small, rounded opacities in the upper lobes with retraction, hilar adenopathy, and "eggshell calcifications."

Epidemiology

Exposure to free silica or crystalline quartz occurs through major occupational hazards such as rock mining, stone cutting, foundry work, quarrying (especially granite), tunneling, sandblasting, pottery making, and packing of silica flour. Progressive pulmonary fibrosis occurs in a dose-response fashion after many years. However, individuals working in small spaces can develop silicosis following periods of exposure as limited as 10 months.

Management

Cessation of silica exposure often necessitates a change in occupation. **Corticosteroids** may improve the chronic lymphocytic alveolitis. Screen for tuberculosis with tuberculin skin test and CXR, as patients with silicosis are clearly at **greater risk of acquiring** *Mycobacterium tuberculosis* (silicotuberculosis) as well as atypical mycobacterial infections.

continued

Multidrug treatment is indicated for any patient with a positive tuberculin test or old, healed tuberculous scars on CXR.

Complications Progressive fibrosis may lead to coalescence of large irregular masses exceeding 1 cm in diameter (progressive massive fibrosis), leading to significant functional impairment with severe **restrictive and obstructive disease** on pulmonary function testing. Respiratory failure may follow within a few years. Atypical silicates such as talc may cause **pleural or lung cancers.**

PULMONARY

TOP SECRET

CASE 48

ID/CC   A 21-year-old male complains of low back pain and stiffness.

HPI   He states that the pain is associated with morning stiffness that gradually improves with exercise. He also complains of fatigue, weight loss, and hip and shoulder pain.

PE   VS: low-grade fever. PE: pallor; stooped posture; reduced inspiratory chest excursion; high-pitched, blowing diastolic murmur (aortic insufficiency); prominent abdomen; fixed kyphosis; poor lumbar spinal mobility; loss of lumbar lordosis; sacroiliac joint tenderness.

Labs   CBC: anemia (Hct 30%). Low serum iron and TIBC (anemia of chronic disease); elevated ESR and C-reactive protein; elevated IgA; negative rheumatoid factor and ANA; positive HLA-B27.

Imaging   [Fig. 48A] XR: periarticular sclerosis with blurred sacroiliac joint margins. [Fig. 48B] XR, spine: ankylosis and fusion of spinal vertebral bodies (BAMBOO SPINE) and sacroiliac joints.

Figure 48A   Figure 48B

continued

Pathogenesis

Ankylosing spondylitis (AS) is characterized by the presence of **inflammatory arthritis** of the **axial skeleton** (classically **sacroiliitis**) that may be accompanied by **peripheral arthritis, enthesitis** (inflammation at the site of tendinous or ligamentous attachment to bone), recurrent acute anterior **uveitis, aortic valve incompetence**, or pulmonary fibrosis. The precise etiology is unknown, but **immune-mediated mechanisms** are likely given the close association with HLA-B27, elevated serum levels of IgA and acute phase reactants, and an inflammatory histology. There is a significant association of AS with inflammatory bowel disease.

Epidemiology

AS usually begins in the second to third decade, is three times more common in **males** than in females, and is more prevalent among first-degree relatives who inherit the B27 allele.

Management

NSAIDs (e.g., indomethacin) are the first line of therapy. Patients must **eliminate cigarette smoking**, initiate a **physical therapy** and **exercise** regimen, receive **genetic counseling**, and minimize spinal trauma to prevent fractures. Anti–tumor necrosis factor drugs (e.g., etanercept or infliximab) are useful in the management of refractory cases. Other immunosuppressants and corticosteroids are of limited or no utility.

Complications

Complications include **spinal fractures and spondylodiscitis** after minimal trauma, and **hip and knee deterioration** necessitating hip or knee replacement. Patients with long-standing disease may develop **aortic insufficiency, conduction defects**, deteriorating vision secondary to recurrent **uveitis** (40% of cases), pulmonary fibrosis, or chronic prostatitis.

RHEUMATOLOGY

ID/CC   A 45-year-old female complains of chronic progressive **muscle weakness** and **tenderness** associated with a diffuse **rash**.

HPI   She is now unable to get up from a sitting position and also has **difficulty raising her arms and climbing stairs** (proximal muscle weakness). She also complains of difficulty swallowing (DYSPHAGIA).

PE   PE: diffuse erythema over the face, neck, shoulders, and upper chest/back (SHAWL SIGN) and maculopapular eruptions; scaly patches over dorsum of PIP and metacarpal joints (GOTTRON'S SIGN); **lilac-colored** rash on eyelids (HELIOTROPE) with periorbital edema; decreased strength in proximal muscle groups.

Labs   Markedly **elevated CK; elevated aldolase**; elevated ESR. UA: myoglobinuria. EMG: low amplitude, short duration motor unit action potentials. Muscle biopsy shows **inflammation** and muscle fiber **necrosis**.

Imaging   XR, soft tissues: diffuse soft tissue calcifications.

Pathogenesis   Dermatomyositis is characterized by the presence of **polymyositis** in association with characteristic **skin changes**. Profound proximal muscle weakness, dysphagia, **respiratory impairment**, and **myocarditis** are key characteristics. The precise etiology is unknown, although viral infection, genetic factors, and autoimmunity are thought to be contributory mechanisms. Polymyositis/dermatomyositis may occur in **association with neoplasia** (breast, gynecologic, or rectal), vasculitis, or other connective tissue diseases (usually progressive systemic sclerosis, rheumatoid arthritis, mixed connective tissue disease, and SLE).

Epidemiology   May develop at any age, with a peak incidence between the fifth and sixth decades of life; **females outnumber males** by a ratio of 2 to 1. The 5-year survival rate is approximately 75%. Poor prognostic factors include delayed treatment, severe disease at initial presentation, underlying malignancy, associated connective tissue diseases, and the presence of antibodies to Jo-1 and signal recognition peptide.

Management   **Corticosteroids** are first-line agents; with improvement beginning as early as 1 to 4 weeks following the initiation of treatment. Measure progress with **serum enzymes. Cytotoxic drugs** (cyclophosphamide, methotrexate, and cyclosporine) may be used in refractory disease. Strength exercises and physical therapy are critical once control of the disease process is established.

Complications   Death may result from cardiac, pulmonary, or renal complications. Patients may have persistent muscle weakness, atrophy, or contracture.

CASE 50

ID/CC

A 45-year-old male presents to the clinic complaining of **severe pain in the right big toe.**

HPI

He states that he has had similar attacks in the past, each of which came on suddenly.

PE

VS: low-grade fever (38.3°C). PE: **tophi** in helix of ear and in hands and feet; **olecranon bursitis** bilaterally; **exquisitely tender, erythematous, swollen, shiny, and warm right first MTP joint** (PODAGRA).

Labs

Serum **uric acid elevated**; synovial fluid aspiration reveals **negatively birefringent crystals** and elevated WBC (20,000).

Imaging

XR, foot: **punched-out erosions of bone** and **overhanging edge of new bone** at the MTP joint of the big toe. XR, hand: soft tissue swelling (due to tophus) of the PIP joint of the index finger.

Pathogenesis

Gout is characterized by the presence of hyperuricemia with resultant **arthritis** (usually monoarticular/inflammatory and presenting as repetitive acute episodes), **tophaceous deposition** in peri- and intra-articular locations, **urate nephropathy** (due to urate crystal deposition in interstitial renal parenchyma), and **nephrolithiasis.** Hyperuricemia may result from **increased dietary intake** of purines in foods such as liver and kidney; **increased de novo synthesis** of purines due to increased activity of PRPP synthetase enzyme; increased breakdown of purines into uric acid due to a **deficiency of HGPRT**-mediated nucleotide salvage mechanism, as in Lesch–Nyhan syndrome; **accelerated purine nucleotide degradation** associated with conditions of rapid cell turnover (tumor lysis syndrome, myeloproliferative diseases, hemolysis, or rhabdomyolysis); or **undersecretion** (most individuals with gout have **defective uric acid clearance**). In acute gout, elevated uric acid levels lead to the development of microtophi, which are shed into the joint space and are subsequently coated by immunoglobulins and complement, promoting phagocytosis by neutrophils. The crystals disrupt the phagosomal membranes, causing lysosomal enzyme release into the joint space and enhancing inflammation.

Epidemiology

Gout arises primarily in **middle-aged and elderly men, postmenopausal women,** and patients with **end-stage renal disease.** Gout is seen more frequently with obesity, diabetes mellitus, hypertension, type II and type IV hyperlipidemia, and atherosclerosis. Additionally, gout may be precipitated by surgery, illness, or excessive alcohol consumption.

Management

Colchicine, NSAIDs, or **intra-articular glucocorticoids** for acute attacks; **allopurinol prophylaxis and uricosuric drugs (probenecid)** for chronic hyperuricemia. Encourage patients to avoid alcohol (inhibits urate excretion) and foods high in purines (e.g., shellfish).

Complications

Nephrolithiasis, renal impairment, destructive arthropathy, and GI bleeding (secondary to high-dose NSAIDs).

RHEUMATOLOGY

CASE 51

ID/CC   A 52-year-old male complains of **weight loss, malaise,** fatigue, headache, and **muscle pain** of 6 months' duration.

HPI   He has no significant past medical history.

PE   VS: **fever** (38.5°C); hypertension (BP 178/95). PE: mild pallor; **diffuse palpable purpura.**

Labs   CBC: anemia (Hct 33%); leukocytosis (13,000); **thrombocytosis;** no eosinophilia. Elevated ESR; hypergammaglobulinemia; **positive hepatitis B surface antigen.** UA: mild **proteinuria;** hematuria; **cellular casts.** Biopsy shows **necrotizing inflammation of small and medium-size arteries.**

Imaging   [**Fig. 51**] Angio, abdominal: **multiple aneurysms of small and medium-size blood vessels.**

Pathogenesis Polyarteritis nodosa is characterized by **necrotizing inflammation of small and medium-sized** arteries (such as renal and visceral arteries). PMN **infiltrates** are prevalent in the **acute stage** of the disease, whereas **mononuclear infiltrates** mark the **chronic stage** of illness. Fibrinoid necrosis later compromises the lumen, causing aneurysmal dilatation, thrombosis, and subsequent infarction of the tissues. Clinical manifestations indicate the organ system involvement: glomerular arteriolitis may

Figure 51

continued

present as hypertension and azotemia; vasa nervorum (arteries supplying nerves) involvement may present as mononeuritis multiplex; and cardiac involvement may present as MI or CHF. The frequent presence of hepatitis B surface antigen suggests an immunologic component.

Epidemiology

A relatively uncommon illness that **presents between the fourth and fifth decades** and affects males and females equally. Associations have been found with SLE, rheumatoid arthritis, hepatitis B virus infection, hairy cell leukemia, and serous otitis media.

Management

Prednisone in combination with **cyclophosphamide** has been shown to be effective. Early initiation of treatment is key. The **control of hypertension** is critical for reducing the morbidity and mortality of cardiac, renal, and CNS complications.

Complications

Death usually results from renal failure, GI complications (bowel infarct), and cardiovascular manifestations. Untreated polyarteritis nodosa has a 100% mortality rate.

RHEUMATOLOGY

ID/CC   A 36-year-old **male** complains of **swelling and pain** in the right **knee** and left **ankle** for the past 2 weeks.

HPI   He reports having suffered a severe case of *Salmonella* **enterocolitis** approximately 1 month ago. He also has **burning on urination** (due to urethritis), irritated eyes, occasional fever, and **moderate weight loss.**

PE   VS: **fever** (38.6°C). PE: mild clear, watery **conjunctival discharge**; mild **stomatitis**; tenderness to palpation, swelling, and erythema in right knee and left ankle with slight effusion.

Labs   CBC/Lytes: normal. **ESR moderately elevated; RA factor negative**; synovial fluid culture negative; positive **HLA-B27.**

Imaging   XR: permanent or progressive joint disease in peripheral joints (articular soft tissue swelling, joint space narrowing, marginal erosions) and in sacroiliac joints.

Pathogenesis   Reiter's syndrome is characterized by the presence of **asymmetric** "**reactive arthritis**" (affecting large weight-bearing joints such as the knees and ankles or **sacroiliitis**), **conjunctivitis** or **uveitis**, **urethritis** (commonly a nongonococcal venereal infection), and **mucocutaneous lesions** (such as balanitis, stomatitis, and keratoderma blennorrhagicum). The presence of **HLA-B27** and characteristic x-ray findings are highly suggestive of the diagnosis of Reiter's syndrome.

Epidemiology   Affects men and women equally following a dysenteric infection (*Salmonella, Shigella, Yersinia, Campylobacter*) or primarily males following an STD (*Chlamydia trachomatis* or *Ureaplasma urealyticum*) within the previous months. Classified as a form of reactive arthritis.

Management   NSAIDs for symptomatic relief. Use **corticosteroids** as needed. It is not known if antibiotics are effective in preventing this syndrome; however, it has been shown that prompt antibiotic administration for chlamydial urethritis may be beneficial. **Tetracycline** used for 3 months may reduce symptom duration and is particularly useful owing to its combination of antimicrobial and anti-inflammatory effects. **Sulfasalazine** is used for patients who are unresponsive to NSAIDs and antibiotic regimens.

Complications   Complications include urethral strictures, permanent joint damage, cataracts, carditis, aortic regurgitation, and **aortic root dissection.** Relapse is common.

ID/CC	A 45-year-old **woman** complains of **vague pain and stiffness** in her **wrists** and **hands** for the past several years.
HPI	Her pain is most **prominent in the morning**, with stiffness typically lasting for more than 1 hour. She reports that her symptoms have progressed, as manifested by the formation of "bumps" (RHEUMATOID NODULES) on her **fingers, wrists,** and **elbows.** She additionally notes increased malaise, weight loss, and generalized weakness.
PE	VS: normal. PE: extremities with decreased range of motion and swelling around **bilateral PIP and MCP joints**; flexion of DIP with extension of PIP (SWAN-NECK DEFORMITY); mild effusion and tenderness in both ankles; [**Fig. 53A**] ulnar deviation of digits at MCP joints with relative sparing of DIP joints; subcutaneous nodules over bony prominences; hyperextension of DIP with flexion of PIP (BOUTONNIERE DEFORMITY); subcutaneous nodules on both elbows.
Labs	CBC: normocytic, normochromic anemia; slight elevation in WBC and platelet counts. ESR moderately elevated; positive **rheumatoid factor**; elevated C-reactive protein; joint fluid with moderate elevation in WBC count (5,000 to 50,000/μL) and > 50% PMNs on differential; negative culture.
Imaging	[**Fig. 53B**] XR, hand: **periarticular osteoporosis** with **erosions** around the affected MCP and PIP joints. [**Fig. 53C**] Another case, more advanced, demonstrates arthritis mutilans, including ulnar deviation of the fingers and carpal fusion.
Pathogenesis	Rheumatoid arthritis (RA) is a chronic inflammatory disorder of **auto-immune** origin that is characterized by **synovitis of multiple joints** with **pannus formation.** Granulation tissue eventually erodes the cartilage, bone, ligaments, and tendons; scarring, contracture, and deformity result from inflammatory destruction of these structures. Any joint may be involved, but the **PIP, MCP, wrists, knees, ankles,** and **toes** are most commonly affected.
Epidemiology	Rheumatoid arthritis is a common disease that **affects females three times more often than males.** The age of onset is usually 20 to 40 years, with prevalence increasing with age, although RA may present at any age. A strong association with **HLA-DR4** has been observed.
Management	**Aspirins/NSAIDs** are first-line therapy unless contraindicated. If these treatment modalities are unsuccessful, **immunosuppressive agents** such as methotrexate, gold salts, hydroxychloroquine, sulfasalazine, or azathioprine may be tried. Tumor necrosis factor inhibitors may be used in patients who have not responded to methotrexate. Oral corticosteroids

RHEUMATOLOGY

should be reserved for unresponsive cases, extra-articular disease or to relieve symptoms while waiting for the effect of immunosuppressive agents. Intra-articular corticosteroids may be tried when only one or two joints are inflamed. Key **nonpharmacologic measures** include weight loss, education, exercise, and assistive devices.

Complications   Complications include **atlantoaxial dislocation**, pleuropulmonary disease (**pleural effusion, pulmonary nodules, Caplan's syndrome**), pericarditis, **Felty's syndrome** (RA associated with splenomegaly and neutropenia), **vasculitis**, and pharmacologic therapy-related side effects (e.g., **aspirin/NSAID-induced GI hemorrhage**). Factors associated with premature death include long length of disease, prolonged steroid use, early age at diagnosis, and low socioeconomic status.

Figure 53A

Figure 53B

Figure 53C

ID/CC

A **34-year-old female** presents to her physician with a **butterfly-shaped rash** over the bridge of her nose and cheeks that is **made worse by sunlight** (PHOTOSENSITIVITY).

HPI

The patient states that she has been experiencing increasing **malaise, fatigue, shortness of breath,** muscle aches, **joint pain,** swelling, and early-morning stiffness over the past 2 months.

PE

VS: fever (38.9°C). PE: diffuse **maculopapular rash** over arms, back, and chest; raised, erythematous **malar rash** over cheeks and nose, extending to ears; **painless oral ulcers;** movements of knees, wrists, and joints of the hands are restricted and painful.

Labs

CBC: normocytic, normochromic anemia; leukopenia. **ANA positive;** elevated ESR; **anti-Sm and anti-dsDNA antibodies** detected; serum C2, C4 complement factors decreased. UA: proteinuria; hematuria; cellular casts (due to lupus **nephritis**).

Imaging

CXR: small right **pleural effusion.** Echo: no signs of pericarditis or pericardial effusion.

Pathogenesis

Systemic lupus erythematosus (SLE) is a disease of unknown etiology in which cells and tissues are damaged by **immune complexes** and **auto-antibodies.** Lack of suppression by typical immunoregulatory systems produces **abnormal hyperactivity** of T and B cells. It is thought that genetic susceptibility, sex hormones, and exogenous antigens influence abnormal self-tolerance in these patients and promote immune cell activation. The antigens that stimulate autoantibodies are both **endogenous** and **exogenous.** Criteria for the diagnosis of SLE include **any four** of the following manifestations: malar rash, discoid rash, photosensitivity, oral ulcers, arthritis, serositis, ANAs, or renal, neurologic, hematologic, and immunologic disorders. The diagnosis of SLE can only be made after drug-induced lupus syndrome has been ruled out.

Epidemiology

Ninety percent of patients with SLE are **women,** typically of **childbearing years.** However, men, children, and the elderly can be affected. Prevalence is higher among **African Americans.** Sex hormones are thought to influence immune tolerance.

Management

Complete remission of SLE is rare. Patients with arthritis, mild pleurisy, and mild pericarditis should be treated with **NSAIDs** only. Use **antimalarial** drugs (retinal damage should be monitored) or **low-dose corticosteroids** for skin and musculoskeletal involvement. Life-threatening or severe SLE should be treated with **high-dose corticosteroids; cytotoxic agents** such as azathioprine, chlorambucil, and cyclophosphamide are

RHEUMATOLOGY

continued

useful for suppression of active disease and lowering the quantity of steroids needed.

Complications Complications include **vasculitic lesions**, including purpura, ulcers, urticaria, and gangrene of the digits; **lupus nephritis**; cognitive dysfunction and seizures with **CNS complications**; ARDS and intra-alveolar hemorrhage; and pancreatitis, abdominal discomfort, diarrhea, vasculitis, and peritonitis. Pericarditis, myocarditis, effusions, arrhythmias, and infarction are manifestations of **cardiac lupus; pleural effusions** may lead to atelectasis, pneumonitis, and infection.

CASE 55

ID/CC

A 42-year-old Caucasian female presents with increasing **sinus pain, bloody nasal discharge,** and **difficulty breathing.**

HPI

The patient adds that she has been experiencing **hemoptysis, shortness of breath,** and general chest discomfort. She also complains of increasing malaise, weakness, loss of appetite, and weight loss. One month ago she started having pain in her left ear with gradual hearing loss and bloody discharge (**otitis media**) that did not respond to a 10-day course of antibiotics.

PE

VS: low-grade fever (38.1°C); tachypnea (RR 24). PE: episcleritis; nasal mucosa ulcerated with bloody discharge; coarse breath sounds bilaterally.

Labs

CBC: leukocytosis and mild anemia. **ESR markedly elevated; antineutrophil cytoplasmic antibodies** (ANCAs; C-ANCA more specific) present; biopsy of lung lesion reveals necrotizing granulomatous vasculitis. UA: **proteinuria** and **hematuria** (secondary to **glomerulonephritis**).

Imaging

CXR: cavitating nodules.

Pathogenesis

Wegener's granulomatosis (WG) is characterized by **granulomatous vasculitis** of the **upper and lower respiratory tracts** with **glomerulonephritis.** Lung involvement appears as multiple, nodular cavitary infiltrates. Upper airway lesions, especially in the sinuses, demonstrate necrosis, inflammation, and granuloma formation.

Epidemiology

WG is a rare disease that affects men and women equally. The disease rarely affects patients before adolescence; mean age of onset is 40 years.

Management

The treatment of choice is **cyclophosphamide** given in combination with **steroids.** WBC count and renal function should be closely monitored. Remissions can be induced in most patients; long-term follow-up is required.

Complications

Focal and segmental glomerulitis may progress into a **rapidly progressive crescentic glomerulonephritis;** nasal ulceration may produce **septal perforation** that may result in **saddle-nose deformity.** Eye complications can produce episcleritis, scleritis, and sclerouveitis.

RHEUMATOLOGY

ANSWER KEY

1. Actinic Keratosis
2. Contact Dermatitis
3. Dermatitis Herpetiformis
4. Erythema Nodosum
5. Kaposi's Sarcoma
6. Psoriasis
7. Seborrheic Dermatitis
8. Squamous Cell Carcinoma
9. Marfan's Syndrome
10. Amebic Liver Abscess
11. Aspergillosis—Allergic
12. Botulism
13. CMV Retinitis
14. Coccidioidomycosis
15. Epidemic Typhus
16. Gonorrhea
17. Herpes Genitalis
18. Herpes Zoster (Shingles)
19. Histoplasmosis
20. Infectious Mononucleosis
21. Legionella Pneumonia
22. Meningococcemia
23. Pneumococcal Pneumonia
24. Rubella (German Measles)
25. Syphilis—Secondary
26. Neurosyphilis (Tabes Dorsalis)
27. Tuberculosis—Pulmonary
28. Typhoid Fever

29. Urinary Tract Infection (UTI)
30. Acute Tubular Necrosis—Ischemic
31. Acute Tubular Necrosis—Toxic
32. Hyperkalemia
33. Membranous Glomerulonephritis
34. Minimal-Change Disease
35. Renal Tubular Acidosis
36. Renovascular Hypertension—
    Fibromuscular Dysplasia
37. Cysticercosis
38. Meningitis—Cryptococcal
39. Septic Arthritis—Staphylococcal
40. Adult Respiratory Distress Syndrome
41. Asbestosis
42. Asthma, Chronic
43. COPD—Chronic Bronchitis
44. COPD—Emphysema
45. Pneumothorax—Spontaneous
46. Sarcoidosis
47. Silicosis
48. Ankylosing Spondylitis
49. Dermatomyositis
50. Gout
51. Polyarteritis Nodosa
52. Reiter's Syndrome
53. Rheumatoid Arthritis
54. Systemic Lupus Erythematosus (SLE)
55. Wegener's Granulomatosis

MINICASES

MINICASE 1: Acne Vulgaris

A common skin disorder caused by excess sebum production and follicular blockage/inflammation

- presents with comedones (follicular cysts) and inflammatory papules, pustules, or nodules, predominantly on the face and trunk
- treat with topical or oral antibiotics, topical keratolytics, or oral isotretinoin (teratogenic) for recalcitrant cases
- the condition usually resolves after adolescence

MINICASE 2: Atopic Dermatitis

An idiopathic, chronic, IgE-mediated skin inflammation

- presents with intense pruritus, lichenification secondary to scratching, erythema, and scaling
- treat with topical corticosteroids, hydrating creams, and removal of potential allergens
- complications include secondary infection

MINICASE 3: Cellulitis

A diffuse, acute spreading infection of the skin involving deeper tissues

- often caused by *Staphylococcus* or *Streptococcus* spp
- presents with pain, redness, swelling, and induration
- treat with cephalexin or dicloxacillin

MINICASE 4: Discoid Lupus Erythematosus

Dermal lupus associated with exposure to solar or UV radiation

- presents with localized erythematous plaques with thick adherent scales, predominantly on the face, scalp, and external ears, along with central scaling, atrophy, and depigmentation
- can cause scarring alopecia
- treat with topical corticosteroids, chloroquine, avoidance of sunlight

MINICASE 5: Dysplastic Nevi

Autosomal-dominant predisposition to develop nevi

- presents with multiple irregular-bordered nevi of pink, tan, and brown shades
- treat with excision if possible and sun protection
- nevi may develop into malignant melanoma

📁 MINICASE 6: Erysipelas

Infection, commonly on the face, by *Streptococcus pyogenes*

- presents with characteristic bright red, raised macule with well-demarcated borders, fever, and pain
- treat with penicillin

📁 MINICASE 7: Erysipeloid

Skin infection caused by *Erysipelothrix rhusiopathiae*, often acquired through contact with fish or swine

- presents with a well-demarcated reddish-purple plaque with severe pain, edema, and induration, usually involving the hand
- isolation of the organism from biopsy or blood is diagnostic
- treat with oral antibiotics (penicillin V, ciprofloxacin)
- rarely complicated by endocarditis

📁 MINICASE 8: Erythroderma

A systemic skin inflammation that is either idiopathic or secondary to underlying dermatologic disease (e.g., psoriasis, dermatitis), cutaneous lymphomas, or drug reactions

- presents with generalized pruritic erythema with lichenification and secondary scaling that may desquamate
- treat with corticosteroids and moisturizers
- treat the underlying condition if it can be determined
- complications include secondary infections, folate deficiency, hypoproteinemia, CHF, dehydration, and sepsis

📁 MINICASE 9: Furuncle

A boil caused by *Staphylococcus aureus* infection of the hair follicle and subcutaneous tissue

- presents with pain, tenderness, and a fluctuant nodule
- treat with incision and drainage followed by penicillinase-resistant antibiotic therapy (e.g., nafcillin)
- risk factors for furunculosis (recurrent furuncles) are IV drug use, diabetes mellitus, and HIV

MINICASE 10: Human Papillomavirus (HPV)—Plantar Warts

Hyperkeratotic lesions on the plantar surface of the foot caused by infection with human papillomavirus (HPV) types 1, 2, or 4

- exposure is often associated with the use of public showers
- presents with foot and heel pain and with yellow-gray, hyperkeratotic lesions
- treat with topical keratolytic agents, cryotherapy, or surgery
- complications include secondary infection and transmission of virus

MINICASE 11: Human Papillomavirus (HPV)—Common Wart

Caused by infection with one of the more than 150 types of HPV

- may affect any area of the skin and mucous membranes and is estimated to occur in 7% to 12% of the world population
- common warts (verruca vulgaris) appear as hard papules with a rough, irregular surface
- diagnosis is usually clinical, but Southern blot hybridization for the HPV DNA is confirmatory
- may spontaneously regress, or treat with topical agents (salicylic acid, cantharidin, dinitrochlorobenzene, dibutyl squaric acid, trichloroacetic acid, or podophyllin), cryosurgery, or lasers

MINICASE 12: Lichen Planus

An inflammatory, pruritic skin disease that is usually idiopathic

- presents with pruritic, violaceous, angulated 1- to 4-mm papules with fine white lines on the wrists, external genitalia, and oral and genital mucous membranes (distributed in a netlike pattern)
- treat with topical glucocorticoids with oral antihistamines for pruritus
- complications include a high rate of recurrence and rare neoplastic degeneration

MINICASE 13: Molluscum Contagiosum

Viral infection of the skin acquired by skin-to-skin contact, often venereal

- common in AIDS patients
- presents with one or more dome-shaped, fleshy papules with central umbilications
- lesions are typically self-limiting
- may treat with cryotherapy

MINICASE 14: Mycosis Fungoides—Sézary Syndrome

The leukemic phase of mycosis fungoides

- usually seen in middle-aged men
- presents with fever, malaise, and erythematous, scaly, extremely pruritic plaques
- Sézary cells seen on PBS
- treat with chemotherapy

MINICASE 15: Osler–Weber–Rendu Disease (Hereditary Telangiectasia)

An autosomal-dominant genetic disorder with abnormal vascular proliferation causing telangiectatic skin lesions, pulmonary AV fistulas, and CNS vascular malformations

- presents with skin and mucosal telangiectases and GI or nasal bleeding
- lab findings include hypochromic microcytic anemia due to iron deficiency
- treat accessible lesions with pressure, styptics, or topical hemostatic agents, iron supplementation for iron deficiency anemia
- complications include brain abscess, ischemic stroke (paradoxical emboli), and severe bleeding episodes

MINICASE 16: Pediculosis

Ectoparasite infestation ("lice") spread by close contact or through fomites

- risk factors include overcrowding, sexual promiscuity, malnourishment, and poor hygiene

- presents with nocturnal itching
- examination reveals small erythematous papules on the back of the head, neck, ears, back, chest, pubic area, and groin
- live parasites fluoresce under Wood's lamp
- treat patients and known contacts by soaking hair in water-vinegar solution, applying permethrin lotion to skin, and washing all clothing and linen
- complications include secondary bacterial infections

MINICASE 17: Pityriasis Rosea

An acute, initially plaque-like exanthem with no known cause

- occurs seasonally, clusters among contacts, and is more common in patients with atopy, seborrheic dermatitis, and acne
- presents with a 1- to 2-cm, scaly, pruritic, salmon-colored herald patch on the trunk, neck, or extremities followed by a secondary eruption of symmetric lesions on the abdomen and thorax in a "Christmas tree pattern"
- skin biopsy is diagnostic
- treatment consists of zinc oxide, calamine lotion, topical steroids, and antihistamines, with refractory cases treated with systemic steroids, dapsone, and UV therapy
- recurrences are rare

MINICASE 18: Pityriasis Versicolor

A common, benign, superficial cutaneous fungal infection caused by the normal skin organism *Malassezia furfur*

- presents with hypopigmented or hyperpigmented macules and patches on the chest and back
- diagnosis is usually clinical, although KOH scraping can confirm cigarbutt hyphae
- treat with topical agents (selenium sulfide or azole antifungals) or oral therapy with antifungals
- complications include recurrence and cosmetic disfigurement

MINICASE 19: Pyoderma Gangrenosum

A large necrotic erosion with heaped-up borders commonly appearing on the shins

- idiopathic but related to ulcerative colitis, Crohn's disease, seronegative spondyloarthropathies
- presents with an acute-onset dark nodule that grows in size and then ulcerates
- treat the underlying disease

MINICASE 20: Seborrheic Keratosis

An idiopathic, benign skin condition of the elderly

- presents with small brown or black skin plaques that appear "stuck on"
- no treatment is necessary
- may be removed with liquid nitrogen for cosmetic reasons

MINICASE 21: Tinea Corporis (Ringworm)

A dermatophyte fungal infection of the skin most often caused by the genera *Trichophyton* or *Microsporum*

- presents with pruritic, annular skin lesions with a raised, advancing, scaly border and central clearing
- KOH stain of scale shows fungal hyphae, culture is confirmatory and most commonly grows *Trichophyton rubrum*
- treat with topical imidazoles, treat widespread or refractory cases with systemic griseofulvin or itraconazole

MINICASE 22: Vitamin A Toxicity

Most often iatrogenic

- presents with alopecia, skin scaling, orange discoloration, papilledema (pseudotumor cerebri), hyperkeratosis, and hepatomegaly
- x-ray of long bones and spine shows subcortical hyperostosis
- treat with moderation of vitamin A intake

MINICASE 23: Vitiligo

Hypopigmentation due to immune-mediated melanocyte destruction that may be idiopathic or associated with systemic autoimmune processes

- presents with patchy, symmetric skin and periorificial depigmentation

- Wood's lamp enhances chalk-white color, biopsy shows minimal inflammation and absence of melanocytes
- treat with glucocorticoids, UV therapy, and grafting

MINICASE 24: Chédiak–Higashi Syndrome

An autosomal-recessive defect of microtubule polymerization leading to impaired chemotaxis, degranulation, and phagocytosis

- presents with recurrent pyogenic staphylococcal and streptococcal infections
- decreased neutrophil count and large cytoplasmic granules
- treat with antibiotics appropriate to the infection

MINICASE 25: Kartagener's Syndrome

An autosomal-recessive disease of defective mucociliary clearance

- presents with chronic cough, recurrent sinusitis, primary sterility, and cardiac apical impulse in the right sixth intercostal space (DEXTROCARDIA)
- CXR shows dextrocardia, saccular and fusiform bronchial dilatation (BRONCHIECTASIS)
- EM shows absence of dynein arms within the cilia of sperm and bronchial cells
- treat with chest physiotherapy, antibiotics, bronchodilators

MINICASE 26: Porphyria Cutanea Tarda

An inherited or sporadic disorder of porphyrin metabolism, associated with alcohol, estrogens, pesticides, and viral hepatitis (HCV)

- presents with painless, fragile skin and blisters on the dorsum of the hands and forearms, skin hyperpigmentation, hypertrichosis, and dark brown urine
- increased uroporphyrin and 7-carboxylate porphyrin in urine, increased isocoproporphyrin in feces, increased total iron-binding capacity, and deficiency of liver uroporphyrinogen decarboxylase
- strongly associated with HCV infection
- treat with phlebotomy, alcohol avoidance, iron supplementation, and low-dose oral chloroquine

📁 MINICASE 27: Actinomycosis

Infection by *Actinomyces israelii*

- presents with abscess of the neck/jaw, abdomen, or chest
- causes classic draining sinuses with "sulfur granules"
- the disease readily crosses tissue planes and invades bone
- biopsy or smear shows branching hyphae-like bacteria
- treat with penicillin

📁 MINICASE 28: Amebiasis

Colonic infection by *Entamoeba histolytica*

- presents with diarrhea with mucus, abdominal cramps, and flatulence
- stool culture reveals causative protozoan
- treat with metronidazole or tinidazole, maintain hydration

📁 MINICASE 29: Aspergillosis

Infection by *Aspergillus* spp, most commonly *Aspergillus fumigatus*

- has three common presentations: allergic bronchopulmonary aspergillosis (ABPA, which presents with cough, dyspnea, fever, and bronchiectasis in chronic cases), aspergillomas (in which the fungus typically colonizes a preexisting cavity from chronic lung disease, tuberculosis, sarcoidosis, or emphysema and presents with hemoptysis), and invasive aspergillosis (bilateral necrotizing bronchopneumonia in patients with prolonged and profound granulocytopenia)

- in ABPA, CBC reveals eosinophilia and the serum precipitating antibody is present, whereas aspergillomas usually yield positive sputum cultures, and invasive aspergillosis is diagnosed on a transbronchial lung biopsy that demonstrates invasion with septate, acute branching hyphae, and positive cultures

- CXR/CT reveal patchy, finger-shaped fleeting infiltrates and later central bronchiectasis in ABPA, whereas aspergilloma is seen as a characteristic intracavitary mass partially surrounded by a crescent of air, and invasive aspergillosis may be seen as a necrotizing bronchopneumonia

- treat ABPA with prednisone and bronchodilators, itraconazole and/or surgical resection for severe hemoptysis with aspergillomas, and amphotericin B/itraconazole for invasive aspergillosis

MINICASE 30: Bacillary Angiomatosis

Skin infection caused by *Bartonella henselae*

- common in HIV infection
- presents with fever and erythematous papules resembling Kaposi's sarcoma
- treat with doxycycline or erythromycin

MINICASE 31: Blastomycosis

Pulmonary or disseminated infection caused by the dimorphic fungus *Blastomyces dermatitidis*

- presents with fever, weight loss, cough, and verrucous skin lesions
- diagnose by blood and sputum cultures, CXR with nodular infiltrates
- treat with amphotericin B

MINICASE 32: Brucellosis

Caused by *Brucella abortus*, a gram-negative, aerobic coccobacillus transmitted to humans by drinking contaminated milk or direct contact with animal tissues

- presents with arthritis and undulating fever
- positive serologies and blood cultures
- treat with doxycycline and gentamicin or streptomycin

MINICASE 33: Chagas' Disease

A parasitic disease endemic to the Americas caused by *Trypanosoma cruzi*

- transmitted by reduviid bug bite
- presents in the acute stage with swollen eyelid from bite (ROMAÑA'S SIGN), ipsilateral auricular and cervical lymphadenitis, fever, and myocarditis
- the chronic stage presents with dilated cardiomyopathy (producing CHF and arrhythmias), megaesophagus (producing dysphagia and regurgitation), and megacolon (producing constipation)
- thick blood smear shows trypanosomes in the acute stage
- positive xenoculture, hemoculture, and serologic tests during the chronic stage
- treat with nifurtimox for acute disease

📁 MINICASE 34: Chlamydia Pneumonia

Caused by *Chlamydia pneumoniae*

- presents with productive cough, few wheezes, and dyspnea
- CXR shows diffuse interstitial infiltrate
- treat with erythromycin

📁 MINICASE 35: Coxsackievirus Infections

Viral syndromes include hand, foot, and mouth disease and aseptic meningitis

- present with malaise, fever, flulike symptoms, and possibly hand and oral ulcerations
- there is no effective treatment
- complications include pericarditis and cardiomyopathy

📁 MINICASE 36: Cryptosporidiosis

Caused by *Cryptosporidium parvum*

- presents as profuse, nonbloody, watery diarrhea, usually in AIDS patients
- acid-fast staining demonstrates oocysts in fresh stool
- treat with fluid and electrolyte repletion
- AIDS patients should boil their water at home to prevent disease contraction

📁 MINICASE 37: Echinococcosis

A zoonosis produced by *Echinococcus granulosus*

- acquired by ingestion of food contaminated with dog feces
- presents with fever and hepatomegaly
- liver cysts can be seen on CT
- treat with surgical drainage
- complications include anaphylaxis resulting from cyst rupture

📁 MINICASE 38: Ehrlichiosis

Infection by tick-borne bacteria of *Ehrlichia* spp

- presents with fever, malaise, myalgia, rash, headache, nausea, and vomiting
- can cause severe pulmonary and CNS disease

- leukopenia and thrombocytopenia
- serologic confirmation by elevated antibody titer on indirect immuno-fluorescence
- treat with doxycycline
- complications include seizures and coma

📁 MINICASE 39: Epidemic Typhus

An infectious febrile illness caused by *Rickettsia prowazekii*

- presents with severe headache, fever, chills, and a macular rash on the trunk and extremities with sparing of the face, palms, and soles
- positive Weil–Felix reaction, rise in complement-fixing antibodies for *R. prowazekii*
- treat with supportive care and antibiotics (tetracycline or chloramphenicol)

📁 MINICASE 40: Gentamicin Side Effects

Aminoglycoside antibiotics can cause nephrotoxicity (acute tubular necrosis) and ototoxicity

- presents with hearing loss, vertigo, and oliguric renal failure
- elevated BUN and creatinine
- granular and epithelial cell casts
- treat by discontinuing drug, giving IV fluids
- ototoxicity may be irreversible

📁 MINICASE 41: Giardiasis

The most common protozoal infection in children in the United States

- transmitted through contaminated food or water
- presents as an acute or chronic diarrhea (bulky, frothy, malodorous, greasy stools) associated with crampy abdominal pain and flatulence, or may present as a malabsorption syndrome
- binucleate, pear-shaped, flagellated trophozoites and cysts found in stool or duodenal fluid sample
- treat with metronidazole

MINICASE 42: Granuloma Inguinale

A chronic ulcerative STD involving the genitals and perineum caused by *Calymmatobacterium granulomatis*

- also called donovanosis

- Donovan bodies (dark-staining, encapsulated, intracellular rod-shaped inclusions in macrophages) demonstrated in crush preparations or fixed tissue sections

- culture of ulceration reveals the organism

- treat with Bactrim, tetracycline, or erythromycin

MINICASE 43: Herpangina

An infection caused by coxsackievirus group A

- presents with sudden-onset high fever of short duration, headache, vomiting, myalgias, sore throat, and characteristic vesicular lesions on the soft palate, tonsils, and pharynx

- CBC reveals mild leukocytosis

- coxsackievirus A isolated from mucosal lesions

- treat with hydration, supportive care

MINICASE 44: Herpes Labialis

Herpes labialis is an extremely common contagious disease infection caused by the herpes simplex virus type 1 (HSV-1) and is characterized by the eruption of small and usually painful blisters on the lips, mouth, gums, or perioral skin

- an extremely common contagious disease that is transmitted through direct or indirect contact

- presents with itching, burning, or a tingling sensation for up to 2 days before characteristic vesicles filled with clear yellowish fluid appear on a red, painful skin area on the lips, mouth, gums, or skin around the mouth

- diagnosis is usually clinical, but a Tzanck test may reveal acantholytic giant cells

- treat with oral acyclovir (may shorten the course of the symptoms)

- complications include recurrences (secondary to reactivation), herpetic keratitis, and dissemination in immune-compromised patients

MINICASE 45: HIV/AIDS

Acquired immune deficiency syndrome is caused by HIV, a retrovirus with a high affinity for CD4 T lymphocytes and monocytes

- acquired through sexual contact, IV drug use, blood products, perinatal transmission, and occupational exposure

- causes profound immunosuppression, rendering the host susceptible to opportunistic infections

- acute HIV presents with flulike symptoms of fever, sore throat, lymphadenopathy, diarrhea, rash, and weight loss

- acute illness is followed by a latent period in which the virus is held in check

- as CD4 count falls below 200, opportunistic infections (*Pneumocystis carinii*, *Mycobacterium tuberculosis*, *Mycobacterium avium*, toxoplasmosis, candidiasis, herpes zoster) may present

- CBC shows lymphocytopenia with a decreased CD4/CD8 ratio

- HIV is diagnosed with ELISA and confirmed with Western blot

- therapy centers on inhibiting viral replication (current regimens include two nucleoside reverse transcriptase inhibitors plus either a protease inhibitor or a non-nucleoside reverse transcriptase inhibitor), antimicrobial prophylaxis, and treatment of opportunistic infections

- complications include opportunistic infections, malignancies, and neuropsychiatric symptoms

MINICASE 46: Human Bite

Usually due to closed-fist injury, chomping injury, or puncture-type injury resulting in direct bacterial contamination that is difficult to treat with normal cleansing

- physical exam reveals the bite wound, which may be overtly infected

- wound culture may reveal bacterial flora of the mouth and skin

- treat with ampicillin and tetanus immune globulin and/or toxoid

- complications include serious soft tissue infection, tendon damage, contracture, osteomyelitis, and cosmetic deformity

MINICASE 47: Influenza

Infection with influenza virus, transmitted via respiratory droplets

- presents with abrupt onset of fever, chills, malaise, cough, coryza, myalgia, and pharyngeal erythema
- CBC may show leukopenia
- viral culture of throat washings, complement fixation, and hemagglutination-inhibiting antibodies are positive for influenza virus
- treat with bed rest, analgesics, antitussives, amantadine
- trivalent virus vaccine confers partial immunity in most cases
- complications include bacterial superinfection, Reye's syndrome in children

MINICAS 48: Leishmaniasis—Visceral

Infection caused by *Leishmania donovani*, transmitted by the sand fly vector

- the disease is endemic in northeastern India, Nepal, and Sudan
- presents with ulcerating lesions in the skin and mucosa of the nasopharynx, darkening of the skin (HYPERPIGMENTATION), and massive splenomegaly
- CBC/PBS show anemia, leukopenia, and thrombocytopenia (PANCYTOPENIA), amastigotes in buffy coat, and Leishman-Donovan (LD) bodies on lymph node and splenic biopsy
- treat with sodium stibogluconate
- high mortality if left untreated

MINICASE 49: Leprosy

Protean infection caused by *Mycobacterium leprae*, most commonly causing disease in Africa and Latin America

- presents with peripheral neuropathies, rashes, peripheral joint and digit destruction, destruction of ear pinna, and hair loss
- biopsy demonstrates acid-fast bacilli
- treat with dapsone and rifampin

MINICASE 50: Lymphogranuloma Venereum

An STD caused by *Chlamydia trachomatis*

- presents with tender inguinal lymphadenopathy, a double genitocrural fold ("groove sign"), and painful genital ulcers

- inguinal node aspirate is diagnostic
- positive immunofluorescence test
- treat with doxycycline or erythromycin

MINICASE 51: Malaria

Plasmodium infection transmitted by mosquitos

- presents with high cyclical fever, fatigue, headache, hepatosplenomegaly, and thrombocytopenia
- plasmodia seen in erythrocytes on peripheral smear
- treat with chloroquine or mefloquine (in resistant areas)
- *Plasmodium falciparum* may lead to lethal cerebral malaria

MINICASE 52: Mycoplasma Pneumonia

The primary cause of "walking" or atypical pneumonia

- presents with fever, sore throat, headache, chills, and nonproductive to minimally productive cough
- associated with extrapulmonary manifestations such as bullous myringitis, cold antibody hemolytic anemia, erythema multiforme, and Raynaud's syndrome
- fourfold rise in complement fixation titer in paired sera, elevated cold-agglutinin titer
- CXR reveals patchy alveolar infiltrates commonly involving the right lower lobe
- treat with erythromycin
- complications include encephalitis, myocarditis, and hemolytic anemia

MINICASE 53: Proctocolitis

Infection of the rectum and colon, commonly by STDs following anal intercourse

- presents with severe rectal pain and blood or mucus per rectum
- endoscopic examination reveals erythema and inflamed rectal mucosa
- treat with doxycycline or Bactrim, sitz baths

MINICASE 54: Pyogenic Granuloma

A polypoid form of capillary hemangioma that occurs as a rapidly growing exophytic red nodule attached by a stalk to the skin or gingival mucosa

- may be related to trauma or to the hormonal changes of pregnancy
- presents with a solitary reddish-brown nodular mass (2 to 3 cm) that may be ulcerated and tends to bleed easily
- biopsy reveals endothelial lined vascular spaces with acute and chronic inflammatory cells but no true granuloma formation
- treat with excisional biopsy
- complications include recurrence

MINICASE 55: Q Fever

A zoonotic infection by *Coxiella burnetii*

- transmitted by livestock
- presents with fever and flulike symptoms
- CXR may show pneumonia
- diagnosis is made with serum serologies
- treat with doxycycline
- chronic Q fever can lead to endocarditis

MINICASE 56: Scabies

A contagious disease caused by infestation of the skin by the mite *Sarcoptes scabiei*

- presents with intense itching that worsens at night and with papulovesicular lesions seen on the finger webs, hands, wrists, elbows, feet, buttocks, and axillae or nodules on the penile glans and shaft
- careful skin scrapings reveal ectoparasite under light microscope
- treat the patient and all family members with 5% permethrin cream or benzyl benzoate or with single-dose ivermectin when topical application is contraindicated

MINICASE 57: Scarlet Fever

Group A β-hemolytic streptococcal infection due to hypersensitivity to erythrogenic toxin

- presents with fever, an extensive erythematous rash, strawberry tongue, and pharyngitis
- culture of throat swab shows *Streptococcus pyogenes*
- ASO titer elevated
- treat with penicillin

MINICASE 58: Shigellosis

Caused by *Shigella* enterotoxin, which activates adenylate cyclase

- presents with nausea, vomiting, and dysentery
- stool exam reveals leukocytes
- stool culture isolates nonmotile *Shigella* bacterium
- treat with rehydration and fluoroquinolones
- complications include Reiter's syndrome and hemolytic-uremic syndrome (following *Shigella dysenteriae* infection)

MINICASE 59: Syphilis—Primary

An STD caused by *Treponema pallidum*, a spirochete

- presents with an indurated, painless chancre and inguinal adenopathy
- treponemes seen on dark-field examination of exudate from chancre
- VDRL positive, FTA-ABS positive
- treat with benzathine penicillin complications
- include progression to secondary or tertiary syphilis if left untreated

MINICASE 60: Syphilis—Tertiary (Aortitis)

Erosion of the aortic intima caused by tertiary syphilitic gummas leading to local dilatation of the aortic root or proximal artery

- presents with aortic regurgitation or can be asymptomatic
- FTA-ABS and VDRL document syphilis, US or CT demonstrates aortic dilatation
- management is surgical correction of the aneurysm and high-dose penicillin to treat the tertiary syphilis
- complications include aortic rupture leading to rapid hemodynamic collapse and death

MINICASE 61: Toxoplasmosis

A systemic disease caused by the parasite *Toxoplasma gondii*

- acquired via cat feces
- common in AIDS patients but can be vertically transmitted
- presents with generalized lymphadenopathy, seizures, and cerebral abscesses (common in immune-compromised patients) and chorioretinitis (the most common manifestation of congenital infection)
- CT shows ring-enhancing brain lesions
- treat with pyrimethamine, sulfadiazine
- AIDS patients receive prophylactic Bactrim

MINICASE 62: Trichinosis

Infection due to *Trichinella spiralis*, acquired by the ingestion of viable larvae in raw or undercooked meat

- presents with myalgias, fever, weakness, diarrhea, facial edema (mostly of the eyelids), and headache, but may progress to neurologic and cardiac involvement
- CBC reveals eosinophilia, elevated CPK
- muscle biopsy demonstrates free or encapsulated larvae
- treat with mebendazole and corticosteroids
- complications include meningitis, CHF, nephritis, and pneumonia

MINICASE 63: Tularemia

Caused by *Francisella tularensis*, a nonmotile, aerobic, gram-negative bacillus transmitted by contact with rabbits, squirrels, or tick bites

- presents with fever, ulcer, and adenopathy with suppuration
- diagnosis is made by direct fluorescent antibody staining
- treat with streptomycin and tetracycline

MINICASE 64: Atopy

Idiopathic propensity to IgE-mediated allergic reactions seen in asthmatics and patients with dermatitis

- strong familial inheritance

- presents with rhinitis, asthma, and eczema
- treatment is avoidance of allergic triggers, supportive use of antihistamines, bronchodilators, and topical corticosteroids

MINICASE 65: Bee Sting

The most common cause of death from envenomation in the United States, bee sting can cause a severe anaphylactic reaction from toxin-mediated stimulation of mast cells

- presentation may range from localized pain and edema to urticaria, shortness of breath, anaphylaxis, and syncope
- treatment involves prompt stinger removal, administration of antihistamines, and emergent management of anaphylaxis if present (bronchodilators, corticosteroids, epinephrine, and vascular/respiratory support)
- complications include infections at sting sites, serum sickness, and rebound anaphylaxis

MINICASE 66: Adult Polycystic Kidney Disease

Bilateral massive enlargement of the kidneys with multiple large cysts

- associated with polycystic liver disease, berry aneurysms, and mitral valve prolapse
- the mode of inheritance of the adult form is autosomal dominant, whereas that of the childhood form is autosomal recessive
- presents with pain, hematuria, hypertension, progressive renal failure, and SAH due to rupture of a berry aneurysm
- US reveals hepatic and renal cysts, carotid angiography reveals the presence of berry aneurysms
- treat hypertension, consider kidney transplant

MINICASE 67: Amyloidosis

Systemic deposition of one of several types of proteins within multiple organs

- can be idiopathic
- associated with diseases such as multiple myeloma or secondary to chronic inflammatory processes
- presents with dysfunction of multiple organs, including nephrotic syndrome, cardiomyopathy, hepatomegaly, and hypothyroidism

- biopsy demonstrates apple-green birefringence after Congo red staining of tissues
- treat the underlying cause (e.g., myeloma), consider organ transplant

MINICASE 68: Diabetic Nephropathy

Insidious proteinuria secondary to diabetic microangiopathy

- chronically progresses to glomerulosclerosis after approximately 10 years
- asymptomatic at first and then presents with hematuria, frothy urine (from protein), anasarca, and hypertension
- UA shows protein and fatty casts
- renal biopsy shows increased mesangial matrix and thickened basement membranes
- treat with ACE inhibitors, protein restriction, strict glucose control with insulin

MINICASE 69: Goodpasture's Syndrome

Hemorrhagic alveolitis with nephritis, seen most frequently in young men

- caused by anti-glomerular basement membrane (anti-GBM) antibodies
- presents with hemoptysis, dyspnea, hematuria, and hypertension
- azotemia, oliguria, and hypoxemia; urine exam reveals proteinuria, RBCs, and RBC casts
- renal biopsy reveals necrotizing proliferative glomerulonephritis with crescent formation in > 50% of glomeruli (on light microscopy)
- anti-GBM antibodies found in the serum constitute the diagnostic marker for the disease
- immunofluorescence microscopy reveals characteristic linear IgG deposits in the glomerular basement membrane
- treat with plasma exchange, corticosteroids, cyclophosphamide, and azathioprine

MINICASE 70: IgA Nephropathy (Berger's Disease)

Idiopathic glomerulonephritis associated with upper respiratory or GI infections

- presents with hematuria
- normal C_3 and elevated serum IgA

- urine shows protein and red cell casts
- renal biopsy shows mesangial IgA deposition
- no effective treatment
- few patients progress to chronic renal failure

MINICASE 71: Interstitial Cystitis

A chronic abacterial bladder disorder occurring primarily in women

- presents with frequency, urgency, and suprapubic pain
- cytoscopy may show cystic wall inclusion bodies or ulcers or decreased bladder capacity
- biopsy to rule out dysplasia or carcinoma in situ
- no effective treatment

MINICASE 72: Membranoproliferative Glomerulonephritis (MPGN)

Idiopathic diffuse glomerular disease

- presents with anasarca, hematuria, and hypertension
- elevated BUN and creatinine, hypocomplementemia
- UA shows fatty casts, RBC casts, and proteins
- treat with aspirin
- renal transplant is the only definitive therapy

MINICASE 73: Nephrotic Syndrome

A clinical complex characterized by proteinuria of > 35 g per 173 m^2 per 24 hr (in practice, > 30 to 35 g per 24 hr), hypoalbuminemia, edema, hyperlipidemia, lipiduria, and hypercoagulability

- six entities account for > 90% of cases: minimal change disease (the most common cause in children), focal and segmental glomerulosclerosis, membranous glomerulopathy (the most common cause in adults), membranoproliferative glomerulonephritis, diabetic nephropathy, and amyloidosis
- presents with lower extremity swelling, periorbital edema, and ascites
- renal biopsies show different patterns on light, immunofluorescence, and electron microscopy

- treatment varies depending on subtype
- in general, corticosteroids, cyclophosphamide, azathioprine, or cyclosporine may be used
- ascites is treated with fluid and salt restriction and diuretics
- renal transplantation should be considered for severe disease or for end-stage renal disease

⬤ MINICASE 74: Renal Transplant

Indicated for patients with end-stage renal disease when conservative treatment has failed and there are no reversible elements to the renal failure

- following a transplant, patients may present with complications related to organ rejection or immunosuppression
- clinically, acute organ rejection presents within the first 3 months with decreased urine output, hypertension, elevated creatinine, and leukocytosis
- immunosuppression is greatest within the first 6 months and accounts for the high incidence of opportunistic infections during that time, with CMV being a common pathogen
- key lab studies include UA, CBC, metabolic panel, and cultures
- complications include infection, graft failure, malignancy, liver failure, and hypertension

⬤ MINICASE 75: Vertebrobasilar Insufficiency

Any interruption in blood flow to the brainstem, cerebellum, or occipital cortex, most commonly caused by atherosclerosis

- presents with vertigo, visual disturbances, facial numbness or paresthesias, dysphagia, dysarthria, syncope, or hemisensory extremity symptoms
- MR/CT to localize area of infarction
- treat with antiplatelet agents, thrombolytics, or anticoagulants, physical therapy
- complications include syndromes such as lateral and medial medullary infarction, basilar artery syndrome (locked-in state), and a persistent neurovegetative state with basilar occlusion

⬤ MINICASE 76: Alcohol Intoxication

Altered mental status due to alcohol ingestion

- presents with mood lability, impaired judgment, inappropriate aggressive and sexual behavior, nystagmus, ataxia, and slurred speech
- treat with thiamine, folate, and sedation as needed
- complications include withdrawal syndrome with seizure, agitation, and delirium tremens

MINICASE 77: Alcoholic Ketoacidosis

Increased anion-gap acidosis

- distinguish from diabetic ketoacidosis by hypoglycemia
- seen in malnourished alcoholics
- presents with altered mental status, nausea, and vomiting
- anion-gap metabolic acidosis
- treat with IV fluids, thiamine, correct electrolyte abnormalities

MINICASE 78: Bronchiectasis

Dilatation of bronchioles secondary to chronic inflammation

- most commonly seen in chronic infection (e.g., tuberculosis, fungal) or cystic fibrosis
- presents with chronic productive cough, repeated pneumonias, hemoptysis, and crackles on exam
- CXR or CT reveals "honeycombing" and "tram tracking" due to bronchial wall thickening
- treat with aggressive chest physiotherapy, antibiotics for infection, and influenza vaccine
- complications include lung and metastatic abscesses and amyloidosis

MINICASE 79: Churg–Strauss Syndrome

Idiopathic systemic small- and medium-vessel granulomatous vasculitis

- presents with asthma and hypertension
- eosinophilia, elevated BUN and creatinine, and proteinuria
- CXR shows bilateral infiltrates
- treat with corticosteroids

MINICASE 80: Hypersensitivity Pneumonitis

An interstitial lung disease that results from inhalation of organic antigens

- presents with dyspnea, fatigue, dry cough, and fine rales
- CXR shows reticulonodular infiltrates
- PFTs show restrictive pattern
- treat with corticosteroids, avoidance of offending agent

MINICASE 81: Interstitial Lung Disease

Inflammation and fibrosis of the interalveolar spaces of the lung

- can be idiopathic or secondary to granulomatous disease, toxic inhalations, particulate toxins (e.g., asbestos, silica), or collagen vascular disease
- presents with acute or chronic progression of dyspnea and exercise intolerance
- CXR reveals classic "honeycomb" appearance of the lung
- spirometry reveals restrictive pathology (proportionately reduced FEV_1 and FVC, hence normal FEV_1/FVC)
- treatment is directed at the underlying cause; supplemental oxygen
- complications include pulmonary hypertension leading to cor pulmonale

MINICASE 82: Löffler's Syndrome

Eosinophilic pneumonia caused by drugs or parasitic infection

- presents with fever, cough, and dyspnea
- peripheral blood eosinophilia
- pulmonary infiltrates on CXR
- remove offending drug or treat parasitic infection, give corticosteroids if no cause is found

MINICASE 83: Lung Transplant

Indicated for patients with nonmalignant pulmonary disease (pulmonary fibrosis, cystic fibrosis, chronic emphysema, α_1-antitrypsin deficiency, and silicosis) who are unresponsive to conventional treatment and who have a life expectancy of < 1 year

- transplant is grafted just superior to the bifurcation at the carina
- current survival rates are 75% to 90% for 1 year and > 50% beyond 2 years
- complications include those of the pleural space (pneumothorax, hemothorax, chylothorax, empyema), those of the lung parenchyma (acute rejection, pulmonary embolism), opportunistic infections that are common in the early postoperative period (bacterial, viral, fungal, parasitic), and immunosuppression-related complications (often GI, hematologic, and hepatobiliary)

MINICASE 84: Primary Pulmonary Hypertension

An idiopathic increase in pulmonary artery pressure and pulmonary vascular resistance, seen in young women

- presents with progressive dyspnea refractory to oxygen therapy, large "a" wave in JVP, and loud P2
- polycythemia
- ECG shows right axis deviation and right ventricular and atrial hypertrophy
- treat with prostacyclin, calcium channel blockers, adenosine, or nitric oxide
- consider heart-lung transplantation, without which the disease progresses to cor pulmonale

MINICASE 85: Pulmonary Eosinophilia Syndromes

Pneumonia characterized by eosinophilic infiltrates

- can be idiopathic or secondary to parasitic infections (e.g., *Strongyloides*, toxocariasis), drug reactions (e.g., penicillin, sulfa drugs), *Aspergillus* infections, Churg–Strauss vasculitis, or asthma
- presents with dyspnea, fever, sputum production, and wheezing
- serum eosinophilia
- CXR reveals pulmonary infiltrates, atelectasis secondary to mucous plugs, and possibly bronchiectasis in chronic disease
- treat with corticosteroids for severe symptoms, bronchodilators for asthma exacerbation, antibiotics for fungal or parasitic infection

MINICASE 86: α_1-Antitrypsin Deficiency

Variable deficiency of enzyme that inhibits trypsin, elastase, and collagenase, causing proteolytic destruction of lung and liver in variable combinations

- presents with panacinar emphysema or hepatic cirrhosis
- PFTs reveal $FEV_1/FVC < 75\%$
- liver biopsy shows cirrhosis
- treat emphysema with home oxygen, human α_1-trypsin replacement therapy may be indicated in some patients
- only transplant can treat liver disease

MINICASE 87: Baker's Cyst

Cyst arising from the synovial lining of the knee

- commonly associated with rheumatoid arthritis
- presents with painful swelling of the popliteal fossa, often mimicking thrombophlebitis
- treat with NSAIDs and leg elevation, consider triamcinolone injection

MINICASE 88: Behçet's Disease

An idiopathic autoinflammatory disease affecting young adults

- presents with recurrent aphthous ulcers, genital ulcers, and anterior uveitis as well as with rashes and large joint arthritis
- treat with systemic glucocorticoids
- complications include blindness

MINICASE 89: Decompression Sickness

Results from the effects of gas (predominantly nitrogen) bubbles on tissues and cells formed by a rapid reduction in pressure while ascending at the end of a dive

- clinical presentation is divided into three categories: type 1 (mild), type 2 (severe), and arterial gas embolization
- may present with joint pain (bends), pruritus, and a sharply defined area of pallor on the tongue (Liebermeister sign), or may progress to pulmonary symptoms, hypovolemic shock, nervous system involvement, and even death
- treat with 100% oxygen, recompression therapy, hyperbaric oxygen, and hydration

- complications include residual paralysis, myocardial necrosis, and other ischemic injuries

MINICASE 90: Drug-Induced Lupus

A reversible lupus-like syndrome most often caused by procainamide, hydralazine, isoniazid, methyldopa, and quinidine

- presents with malar rash, arthralgias, and pericardial friction rub
- anti-histone antibody positive
- kidneys and CNS are usually spared
- treat by removing the offending agent
- steroids may be used for severe symptoms
- the disease is self-limiting

MINICASE 91: Felty's Syndrome

Systemic rheumatoid arthritis coupled with splenomegaly and neutropenia

- presents with infections, purpura, and splenomegaly
- neutropenia and thrombocytopenia
- abdominal CT demonstrates enlarged spleen
- treat the underlying rheumatoid arthritis, splenectomy may ameliorate disease

MINICASE 92: Mixed Connective Tissue Disorder

An idiopathic syndrome with variable characteristics of SLE, systemic sclerosis, polymyositis, and rheumatoid arthritis

- presents with Raynaud's phenomenon, arthritis, skin disease, and diffuse organ disease
- anti-U1RNP antibodies
- treat with corticosteroids, NSAIDs

MINICASE 93: Osteoporosis

Quantitative reduction of total skeletal bone mass due to increased bone resorption

- usually seen in postmenopausal women (preventable with post-menopausal estrogen replacement)
- commonly presents with spinal compression fractures, wrist fractures, hip fractures, or acquired kyphosis
- DEXA scan reveals diminished bone density
- x-rays of the spine may reveal kyphosis and osteoporotic collapse of mid- to lower thoracic and lumbar vertebrae
- treat with calcium supplements, estrogen, bisphosphonates, and exercise
- complications include fractures, loss of height, kyphosis

MINICASE 94: Polymyalgia Rheumatica

An inflammatory condition whose median age of onset is 70

- female-to-male ratio is 2:1
- associated with HLA-DR4 and giant cell (temporal) arteritis
- presents with aches in the shoulder, hip girdle muscles, and proximal extremities that worsen in the morning
- elevated ESR and normochromic anemia
- treat with corticosteroids

MINICASE 95: Polymyositis

Inflammation of skeletal muscle

- 10% of cases are associated with coexisting malignancy
- presents with progressive proximal muscle weakness with atrophy and associated skin findings in dermatomyositis (heliotrope rash, Gottron's papules, photosensitive skin rash)
- elevated CPK
- EMG and muscle biopsy (showing myonecrosis and perivascular mononuclear infiltrates) are suggestive
- treat with high-dose corticosteroids, methotrexate, seek the underlying malignancy

MINICASE 96: Progressive Systemic Sclerosis (Scleroderma)

An idiopathic autoimmune fibrosing disorder

- presents with diffuse skin fibrosis with telangiectasis, Raynaud's phenomenon, dysphagia, and cardiac and renal problems
- treat with corticosteroids for acute exacerbations
- penicillamine may be helpful

MINICASE 97: Psoriatic Arthritis

Autoimmune arthritis seen in patients with psoriasis

- presents with asymmetric large and small joint arthritis
- commonly affects the DIP joints of the fingers
- waxing and waning course
- patients are often HLA-B27 positive
- treat the underlying skin disease, NSAIDs for arthritis
- complications include severe joint erosions

MINICASE 98: Sjögren's Syndrome

Autoimmune destruction of exocrine glands, often associated with other autoimmune disease (e.g., rheumatoid arthritis, SLE, scleroderma)

- primarily affects middle-aged women
- presents with dry mouth and eyes, parotid enlargement, and denuded corneal epithelium
- hypergammaglobulinemia
- ANA and RF positive
- treatment is supportive (e.g., eye drops)

MINICASE 99: Takayasu's Arteritis

Medium- and large-vessel arteritis

- common in young Asian females
- presents with fatigue, fever, and decreased peripheral pulses
- increased ESR and elevated immunoglobulin levels

- arteriography demonstrates inflammatory aneurysms
- treat with corticosteroids

MINICASE 100: Temporomandibular Joint Syndrome

Believed to be a stress-related disorder caused by grinding of the teeth (BRUXISM), resulting in muscle spasm and pain

- presents with pain and tenderness in the muscles of mastication and in the TMJ as well as with crepitus when the joint is moved, decreased range of motion, headaches, and earaches
- treat with NSAIDs or benzodiazepines
- complications include alterations in dentition, chronic facial pain, and malocclusion

1. A 32-year-old black female presents with a 3-month history of nonproductive cough and dyspnea, especially with climbing stairs. She reports intermittent fevers to 39°C (102°F) and a 3.5 kg weight loss. She reports some pleuritic-type chest pain with cough. She denies hemoptysis, palpitations, and nausea. On further questioning, the patient also complains of wrist and ankle pain, which has interfered with her work as a nursing assistant on the obstetrics ward. She also has red nodules over her lower legs. The patient smokes two packs per day and drinks only on the weekends. Complete blood count is normal, and a serum ANA is negative. What is the most likely diagnosis?

    A. Goodpasture's disease

    B. Histoplasmosis

    C. Systemic lupus erythematosis

    D. Sarcoidosis

    E. Adenocarcinoma of the lung

2. A 17-year-old white female has just moved into the area and is seeking a new primary care provider. She has a history of asthma, for which she has been hospitalized twice in the past. She has never required intubation. She states that she usually needs a burst of steroids for worsening symptoms 3–4 times per year, mainly in the spring and fall. She currently uses an albuterol metered-dose inhaler 2–3 times per day. She also has a nebulizer machine and uses nebulized albuterol and atrovent for acute attacks. Examination reveals a cooperative young woman in no acute distress. Her lungs are clear to auscultation, and her expiratory phase is not prolonged. What is the best change to make to her medical management at this time?

    A. Instruct the patient to use her nebulized albuterol instead of her MDI.

    B. Give the patient a 5-day course of prednisone.

    C. Add theophylline to the patient's daily medical regimen.

    D. Tell the patient to use her metered-dose inhaler four times per day.

    E. Add inhaled beclomethasone to the daily medical regimen.

3. A 45-year-old woman with rheumatoid arthritis presents to the emergency department complaining of right leg pain. She states that she was in her usual state of health yesterday, but that she noticed that her right leg was swollen and painful when she got out of bed this morning. She denies any fevers, rashes, or difficulty breathing. She also denies any recent trips involving long periods of immobility. Her medications include methotrexate, naprosyn, and hydroxychloroquine. On examination, her right leg is considerably larger than the left, and she experiences pain when her foot is passively dorsiflexed. What is the next best step in management of this patient?

    A. Begin a heparin drip.

    B. Obtain a ventilation–perfusion scan to rule out pulmonary embolus.

C. Stop the patient's methotrexate.

D. Obtain an ultrasound with Doppler of the patient's right leg.

E. Order venography of the patient's right leg.

4. A 38-year-old white female presents with complaints of morning stiffness and joint pain in multiple joints. Which of the following does not support the diagnosis of rheumatoid arthritis?

A. Ibuprofen helps to control her pain.

B. The patient has firm nodules palpated on the extensor surfaces of her elbows.

C. The patient has involvement of her MCP and DIP joints bilaterally.

D. Periarticular erosions are seen on x-ray of her wrists.

E. The patient is found to have splenomegaly and leukopenia.

5. A 30-year-old asthmatic is in the intensive care unit with a severe asthma exacerbation. He has been stable on the ventilator for the past 12 hours. The nurse notes that his oxygenation has suddenly dropped. On examination, the patient has diffuse expiratory wheezes on the left and absent breath sounds on the right. The patient's trachea is deviated to the left. The patient appears agitated, and his oxygen saturations have dropped to 84%. What is the most likely cause of this patient's decompensation?

A. The patient has developed a nosocomial pneumonia.

B. The patient's asthma exacerbation has worsened.

C. The patient has a mucous plug occluding the endotracheal tube.

D. The patient has severe atelectasis on the right because of lying flat in bed for so long.

E. The patient has a pneumothorax on the right.

6. A 28-year-old Japanese-American woman is referred by her gynecologist for work-up of hypertension. She has been previously healthy except for some generalized fatigue over the past 6 weeks. She has never been pregnant, and her menstrual periods are regular and without excessive bleeding. On physical exam, the patient is thin and in no acute distress. Her heart rate is 90 with a blood pressure of 150/92. On cardiac exam, she has a diastolic murmur heard best at the left lower sternal border. Radial pulses are very weak bilaterally. There are no rashes or edema. Urinalysis is normal. What is the most likely diagnosis?

A. Takayasu's arteritis

B. Membranoproliferative glomerulonephritis

C. Essential hypertension

D. Spontaneous bacterial endocarditis

E. Buerger's disease

7. A 19-year-old white female presents with a nonproductive cough. She says that the cough has been present for 3 weeks now. She has also noticed some

nasal congestion and says that her eyes get "itchy" in the evenings. She denies shortness of breath, wheezing, fevers, or hemoptysis. She has had similar problems in the past, always in the spring and fall. She has no pets. She smokes half-a-pack of cigarettes per day. On physical exam, the patient is afebrile and is not in respiratory distress. She has mild bilateral conjunctival injection. Her nasal turbinates are boggy and have a bluish tinge. She has mild tenderness to percussion over the maxillary sinuses, and there is a small amount of drainage in her posterior pharynx. Lungs are clear to auscultation bilaterally and without wheezing. What is the most likely cause of her cough?

    A. Acute bronchitis
    B. Smoker's cough
    C. Bacterial sinusitis
    D. Allergic rhinitis
    E. Chronic bronchitis

8.   A 24-year-old male presents to the community health center with acute groin pain. He reports that the pain has been present for 5 hours, and it is so severe that he is unable to walk. He denies dysuria, hematuria, or penile discharge. He has not experienced any trauma to the area. He has a past medical history significant for primary syphilis 2 years ago, but is otherwise healthy. He was treated at that time with IM penicillin. He now has a fever to 101°F. On exam, his left testicle is extremely tender to palpation with associated warmth and swelling. There is a fairly firm tender mass palpated along the posterior aspect of the testis. Cremasteric reflex is intact, and there is no change in the pain with elevation of the scrotum. There are no other abnormal physical findings. Urinalysis is positive for leukocyte esterase. What is the most appropriate therapy?

    A. PO bactrim for 7 days
    B. PO doxycycline and IM ceftriaxone
    C. Transfer to the hospital for immediate surgical consult
    D. IV ceftriaxone for at least 5 days
    E. Referral to urologist for biopsy and probable chemotherapy

9.   A 33-year-old male was seen in the community health center complaining of a rash for the past 3 days. It is maculopapular and involves his trunk, arms, and legs, including his palms and soles. He also reports headache, malaise, and subjective fevers. He has been previously healthy, although he was treated for gonorrhea 1 year ago. He states that he had a "sore" on the shaft of his penis about 2 months ago, but that it resolved spontaneously. He denies any dysuria or penile discharge, but he does complain of a bitemporal headache. He takes no medications. Physical exam reveals the rash described above, a fever of 101°F, and lymphadenopathy in the cervical, axillary, and inguinal regions. There is no nuchal rigidity, and cardiopulmonary exam is normal. What test is most likely to be diagnostic in this patient?

A. Cerebrospinal fluid for gram stain and culture
B. Skin biopsy
C. Urethral swab for culture
D. Blood cultures
E. None of the above

10. A 23-year-old white female presents with a 2-month history of nonproductive cough. The symptoms began shortly after she moved to rural Ohio from Phoenix, Arizona. She reports that her cough is worse at night. She has also noticed some nasal congestion and says that her eyes get "itchy" in the evenings. She denies shortness of breath, wheezing, fevers, or hemoptysis. She has never had such problems before. She has no pets. She works as a school bus driver. When she moved to Ohio in August, she purchased a 100-year-old home on a wooded lot in the country. On physical exam, the patient has mild bilateral conjunctival injection. Her nasal turbinates are boggy and have a bluish tinge. She has mild tenderness to percussion over the maxillary sinuses, and there is a small amount of drainage in her posterior pharynx. Lungs are clear to auscultation bilaterally, and she has no wheezing. What is the next best course of action?

A. Begin therapy with amoxicillin.
B. Treat with oral azithromycin.
C. Instruct the patient to take diphenhydramine as needed to control symptoms.
D. Start therapy with a steroid nasal spray.
E. Send serology for coccidioidomycosis.

11. A 60-year-old female presents with acute onset of knee pain. She reports a 1-day history of pain and decreased movement of her right knee. On exam, she has a fever of 38.0°C (100.4°F). Her knee is tender, erythematous, and swollen with a large effusion. Arthrocentesis results show a WBC count of 60,000/mm^3 and needle-shaped, negatively birefringent crystals. What is the best initial therapy for this patient?

A. Allopurinol
B. Probenecid
C. Broad-spectrum antibiotics
D. Physical therapy to improve joint range-of motion
E. Indomethacin

12. A 44-year-old white male presents for evaluation of "chronic allergies." He explains to you that he has been treated for sinusitis several times a year over the past 3 years. He has also had an intermittent cough, generalized fatigue, and a 3-kg weight loss over the past 6 months. Physical examination of the chest reveals scattered crackles bilaterally. A chest x-ray shows multiple bilateral cavitary lesions, but no hilar adenopathy. Urinalysis shows 2+ blood and 2+ protein. Microscopic examination of the urine shows red cell casts. Which of the following test results is most likely to be seen in this patient?

A. Eosinophilia
B. Positive PPD skin test
C. Positive serum antinuclear antibody
D. Positive c-ANCA
E. Lung biopsy positive for noncaseating granuloma

13. A 40-year-old woman with a history of Crohn's disease sees you for complaints of diffuse bony pain. Her Crohn's disease is not well controlled, and she has frequent loose stools and a 5-pound weight loss over the last 3 months. She has some problems with weakness, and you note mild proximal muscle weakness and a waddling gait. You discover a serum calcium of 8.2 mg/dl (normal range 8.4–10.2), and a serum phosphorus of 2.0 (normal range 3.0–4.5). Skeletal films show multiple pseudofractures and her alkaline phosphatase is twice normal. Appropriate therapy would be:

   A. Vitamin C
   B. Bisphosphonates
   C. Fluoride
   D. Vitamin D
   E. Parathyroidectomy

14. A 40-year-old woman sees you for obesity and skin changes. You note hypertension, truncal obesity, purple striae on her breasts and abdomen, and a fasting blood sugar of 150. In your evaluation for Cushing's syndrome you confirm hypercortisolism by finding a high 24-hour urine free cortisol. You find inadequate suppression of both low-dose and high-dose dexamethasone suppression tests, and an ACTH level is nondetectable. Which procedure would best localize the etiology of Cushing's syndrome?

   A. Chest x-ray
   B. CT scan of the chest
   C. CT scan of the abdomen
   D. MRI of the pituitary
   E. Pelvic ultrasound

15. A 30-year-old man comes to see you with a chief complaint of heartburn for the past three months. He says that he has a burning pain in his chest and upper abdomen that is associated with belching and a "nasty" taste in his mouth. This occurs almost every day and occasionally awakens him at night. He denies weight loss, dysphagia, or vomiting. The patient has smoked for the past 10 years. He drinks "a couple of beers" on the weekends. On physical exam, his abdomen is obese with normal bowel sounds, and there is no tenderness to palpation. His rectal exam is guaiac negative. Which of the following is the appropriate first step in managing this patient's GERD?

   A. Advise the patient to quit smoking cigarettes and drinking alcohol.
   B. Draw an *H. pylori* serology.
   C. Prescribe a promotility agent.

D. Order an upper GI series.

E. Refer to a gastroenterologist for endoscopy.

16. A 20-year-old female nursing assistant is seen in her physician's office in New York City. The day prior to being seen, she returned from a camping trip in Vermont. On the day before she returned home, she noticed a tick crawling on her scalp. She removed the tick, but she did not keep it and is not able to describe it well except that it was dark-brown and small. She is currently asymptomatic, but is worried about getting Lyme disease. This was her first camping trip, and she is not planning to take another such trip soon. Which of the following is the best course of action?

   A. Begin doxycycline 100 mg BID.

   B. Reassure patient and pursue no further workup or therapy.

   C. Send serology for antibody to *Borrelia burgdorferi* and treat if positive.

   D. Give the patient the vaccine for Lyme disease.

   E. Hospitalize patient for IV ceftriaxone.

17. A 42-year-old businessman comes to see his primary care physician for diarrhea. He reports a 2-day history of loose stools 7–8 times per day. He has also had episodic crampy abdominal pain and nausea but no vomiting. He has been previously healthy and takes no medications. He recently returned from a business trip to Mexico City. He is married with two young children, and no one else in his household has been ill. On physical exam, he has a temperature of 37.1°C (98.8°F), pulse of 90, and blood pressure of 126/74 without orthostasis. He has diffuse mild abdominal tenderness without rebound. There is no organomegaly or abdominal masses, and he is not jaundiced. Which of the following is the most likely cause of his symptoms?

   A. *Clostridium difficile*

   B. *Escherichia coli*

   C. *Giardia lamblia*

   D. *Salmonella typhi*

   E. Ulcerative colitis

18. A 29-year-old woman is 15 weeks pregnant with her first child. She comes to the office complaining of 2 days of urinary frequency and dysuria. She denies hematuria, nausea, or back pain. She has been previously healthy, and her pregnancy has been uncomplicated. Exam reveals only mild suprapubic tenderness to palpation. She has no fever and no tenderness to percussion in the costovertebral angles. Urine dipstick reveals 1+ protein, 2+ blood, 1+ nitrites, and 2+ leukocyte esterase. What is the best therapy for this patient?

   A. Oral ciprofloxacin for 3 days

   B. Intravenous ceftriaxone

   C. Amoxicillin for 7 days

   D. Send urine for culture and base therapy on results.

   E. No antibiotic therapy is necessary since this patient is afebrile.

19. A 62-year-old farmer presents with a history of worsening dyspnea and cough over the past 9 months. He has no fever, hemoptysis, wheezing, or weight loss. He noticed that his symptoms improved significantly when he took a trip to Phoenix to visit his daughter, but they worsened when he returned home. The patient notes that he had a positive PPD test 15 years ago for which he received no therapy. He smokes 3–4 cigars a day and takes metoprolol for hypertension. A chest x-ray shows bilateral infiltrates. Pulmonary function tests show a restrictive pattern with decreased gas diffusion. What is the most likely diagnosis?

    A. Hypersensitivity pneumonitis
    B. COPD
    C. Coccidioidomycosis
    D. Reactivation of latent tuberculosis
    E. Drug toxicity

20. A 26-year-old woman presents to your office with extreme progressive dyspnea with even mild exertion over the last several months. The shortness of breath is often associated with chest pain. There is no past history of heart, lung, or connective tissue disease. There is no history or risk factors for DVT or pulmonary embolus. Chest x-ray reveals engorged pulmonary arteries and a cardiac silhouette suggestive of RVH but is otherwise clear. Her EKG is remarkable only for right axis deviation. She is a well-developed, well-nourished young woman who appears pleasant but somewhat anxious about her symptoms. Her lung fields are clear to auscultation, and you detect findings consistent with RVH on cardiac exam, but there are no murmurs. You begin to counsel the patient on her likely diagnosis and the therapies she may need. Which agents should be most prominent in your discussion?

    A. Calcium-channel blockers, anticoagulation with warfarin (Coumadin), and supplemental oxygen
    B. Beta-blockers and anxiolytics
    C. ACE inhibitors, diuretics, and digoxin
    D. Anxiolytics and bedtime antidepressants
    E. Nasal steroids, antihistamines, and decongestants as required

1. **D. This patient has a classic case of sarcoidosis. It is most common in black females. The clinical manifestations typically include a dry cough, arthralgias, and systemic symptoms including fever, weight loss, and fatigue. Erythema nodosum is also frequently seen in patients with sarcoid.**

   A. Goodpasture's disease is an autoimmune disease causing hemoptysis, anemia and diffuse pulmonary infiltrates along with glomerulonephritis.

   B. Histoplasmosis is a fungal infection that is usually subclinical. But in an immunocompromised patient, it may present with pulmonary infiltrates as well as skin and bone marrow involvement.

   C. Although she has both arthritis and symptoms of pleural inflammation, this patient does not have enough symptoms to meet criteria for SLE.

   E. Lung cancer can cause weight loss and pulmonary symptoms, but it does not cause arthralgias or erythema nodosum. Also, this patient is quite young to have lung cancer from her smoking.

2. **E. Inhaled steroids are good maintenance medications for asthma. Daily use of inhaled steroids has been shown to improve symptoms and decrease hospitalizations. This patient has sufficiently frequent symptoms to warrant the addition of inhaled steroids to her daily regimen.**

   A. When used correctly, nebulized albuterol is no more effective than a metered-dose inhaler. However, during an acute attack sometimes tachypnea can prevent a patient from being able to use an MDI properly.

   B. Systemic steroids should be reserved for acute attacks.

   C. Theophylline would not generally be added before an inhaled steroid because of its considerable side effects.

   D. The beta agonists should be used only as often as is needed to keep symptoms under control.

3. **D. This patient had a Baker's cyst behind her right knee that ruptured. A ruptured Baker's cyst (which is relatively common in rheumatoid arthritis) may mimic a DVT. An ultrasound will show the ruptured cyst. A Doppler ultrasound would also diagnose a proximal DVT.**

   A. It is inappropriate to begin heparin prior to diagnosis in this patient who may not have a DVT.

   B. This patient has no symptoms of a pulmonary embolus.

   C. There is no reason to stop this patient's methotrexate.

   E. Venography is not superior to ultrasound in diagnosing DVT, and it will not diagnose a Baker's cyst.

4. **C. Rheumatoid arthritis does not involve the DIP joints. However, the PIPs and MCPs are very frequently involved. RA typically is a symmetric arthritis that includes morning stiffness of more than an hour.**

A. NSAIDs are a very important part of managing the pain of RA.

B. Rheumatoid nodules are one of the diagnostic criteria of RA.

D. This is a typical radiologic finding in a patient with RA.

E. Felty's syndrome consists of rheumatoid arthritis and splenomegaly and leukopenia.

5. **E. This patient has developed a tension pneumothorax on the right side secondary to high ventilatory pressures. This is why he has the absence of breath sounds on the right. Left-sided tracheal deviation is due to increased right-sided intrathoracic pressure from the air in the pleural space.**

A. A nosocomial pneumonia would not account for this sudden change in the patient's status or the tracheal deviation.

B. A worsening of the asthma could cause diminished to absent breath sounds, but would not likely present so acutely, nor would it cause tracheal deviation.

C. A mucous plug, either in the ETT or a bronchus, could cause a sudden worsening in respiratory status, but it would not explain this patient's physical exam findings.

D. If the patient had atelectasis, the trachea should be deviated *toward* the side of diminished breath sounds.

6. **A. This patient has Takayasu's arteritis, a vasculitis affecting mainly the aorta and its major branches. It is most common in young women, and it can involve hypertension from renal artery stenosis and aortic regurgitation from aortitis. Diminished or absent pulses is a classic sign of this disease. Generalized fatigue is also common, and other systemic signs like fevers and elevated ESR can also be seen.**

B. Although glomerulonephritis can cause hypertension, it should include blood and often RBC casts on urinalysis.

C. Essential hypertension is a diagnosis of exclusion. This patient has too many secondary signs to diagnose essential hypertension, including a heart murmur and diminished pulses.

D. Despite this patient's heart murmur, there are no peripheral stigmata of SBE (like Janeway lesions, Osler's nodes, splinter hemorrhages, and Roth spots) and no fever. Furthermore, endocarditis does not cause hypertension.

E. Buerger's disease is a disease of peripheral vascular insufficiency seen in smokers. This is a disease of small vessels and would not cause aortic insufficiency.

7. **D. This patient has classic symptoms of allergic rhinitis with "post-nasal drip." The seasonal nature of her symptoms further supports this diagnosis.**

A. This patient has no fevers, and her cough is nonproductive. Also, the itchy eyes and boggy nasal turbinates are more suggestive of allergic rhinitis than an infectious etiology.

B. A smoker's cough would be unlikely to be seasonal, and it would not account for her eye and nose findings.

C. Despite the mild sinus tenderness, this patient is more likely to have seasonal allergies causing her symptoms and causing some sinus fullness.

E. Chronic bronchitis involves a productive cough for at least 3 months of the year for at least two consecutive years. Furthermore, it generally is seen in older patients with a long smoking history.

8.   **B. This patient has acute epididymitis, most commonly caused by *Chlamydia trachomatis* in a young adult patient, but gonorrhea is another possible etiology. Treatment is with one dose of IM ceftriaxone and oral doxycycline for 14 days. In older patients, the etiology is more commonly gram-negative organisms like those seen in the GI tract.**

A. Although good therapy for a UTI, trimethoprim-sulfamethoxazole does not have good coverage of chlamydia, the most common cause of epididymitis.

C. Testicular torsion, which is in the differential diagnosis of acute groin pain in a young adult male, requires immediate surgery. However, it typically has an absent cremasteric reflex, and pain worsens with elevation of the testicle. Also, it does not typically cause fevers or WBCs in the urine.

D. Epididymitis does not typically require IV antibiotics, and ceftriaxone would not cover chlamydia.

E. Although testicular cancer is seen primarily in young men, it is typically painless. Fever and WBCs in the urine are also not consistent with testicular malignancy.

9.   **E. This patient has secondary syphilis. Classic symptoms include fever with a rash, generalized malaise, headache, and lymphadenopathy. Approximately 25% of patients with primary syphilis who are untreated will develop secondary syphilis, and many will not give a history of the chance of primary syphilis. The initial screening test for syphilis is either the VDRL or the RPR serologic test. If this is positive, it is useful to do a confirmation with the more specific FTA-ABS test for *Treponema pallidum* antigen. Treatment efficacy can be monitored with decrease in VDRL or RPR titers.**

A. Bacterial meningitis can cause fever and headache, but the "rash" associated with meningococcal meningitis is purpuric in nature. Furthermore, this patient had no nuchal rigidity, and his lymphadenopathy would not be seen with meningitis.

B. A skin biopsy is not necessary in this patient. His diagnosis can be made with serology.

C. *Treponema pallidum* cannot be cultured in the laboratory. Diagnosis is made by visualization of the spirochete from moist lesions by means of dark-field microscopy (for primary syphilis) or by serology.

D. Again, *T. pallidum* cannot be cultured in the laboratory.

10. **D. This patient has classic symptoms of allergic rhinitis with "postnasal drip." She is most likely sensitive to something in her new environment. First line therapy is a glucocorticoid nose spray. Antihistamines can also be used, but this patient should be given a nonsedating antihistamine because her job requires alertness.**

A. In this patient with a nonproductive cough and no fevers who has classic symptoms of allergic rhinitis/sinusitis, antibiotics are not indicated.

B. This patient's sinusitis symptoms are most likely secondary only to her allergic rhinitis. Her cough is caused by postnasal drip.

C. Although diphenhydramine would likely help this patient's allergic symptoms, it would also make her drowsy. This would be unsafe in a school bus driver.

E. Although coccidioidomycosis can cause a chronic cough, there is no other clinical evidence of this disease.

11. **E. This patient has acute gout, with uric acid crystals seen in her synovial fluid. Indomethacin is good for treating the pain of an acute attack.**

A. Although allopurinol works to decrease uric acid levels in the serum by blocking xanthine oxidase, it is a poor choice during an acute attack. Abrupt changes in uric acid levels in the setting of an acute gouty flare can exacerbate the symptoms.

B. Probenecid lowers uric acid levels by increasing its excretion in the urine. However, this does not help with the symptoms of an acute attack.

C. The crystals in the synovial fluid make septic arthritis less likely. If this was a septic joint, the target of antibiotic therapy would be gram-positive organisms like *Staphylococcus aureus*.

D. Although physical therapy can be helpful in osteoarthritis and other causes of chronic joint pain, there is little role for it in an acute attack of gout.

12. **D. This patient has Wegener's granulomatosis. This is an inflammatory, necrotic granulomatous disease that mainly involves the lungs, kidneys, and upper respiratory tract (including sinusitis and glomerulonephritis). It does not include hilar adenopathy on chest x-ray. Antineutrophil cytoplasmic antibody is a classic marker supportive of the diagnosis of WG. However, it is not diagnostic because it can be seen with several other autoimmune diseases. Diagnosis is made by biopsy of the lung, nose, or sinuses.**

A. High levels of eosinophils can be seen in several lung conditions, including allergic bronchopulmonary aspergillosis and Churg–

Strauss vasculitis. But these conditions do not typically involve the kidneys or sinuses.

B. Although the cavitary lesions might suggest pulmonary tuberculosis, this condition usually also includes hilar adenopathy. It is rare to include glomerulonephritis and sinusitis.

C. Although ANA is positive in many autoimmune diseases, it is not typically seen with Wegener's granulomatosis.

E. The granulomas of Wegener's disease are necrotic. Noncaseating granulomas are seen with sarcoidosis. This patient does not have symptoms consistent with sarcoid, which classically involves hilar adenopathy and/or pulmonary infiltrates.

13. **D. This patient has Crohn's disease and malabsorption, leading to vitamin D deficiency and osteomalacia. Vitamin D deficiency results in secondary hyperparathyroidism due to decreased abdominal absorption of calcium. The biochemical consequences are low serum calcium and phosphate levels with elevated alkaline phosphatase and PTH levels. Besides treating the Crohn's disease more aggressively, optimal therapy would be vitamin D replacement and appropriate calcium supplementation.**

A. Vitamin C would not help this patient's osteomalacia.

B. Bisphosphanates are inappropriate for osteomalacia due to vitamin D deficiency.

C. Fluoride may be helpful in ancillary therapy for osteoporosis, it has no role in osteomalacia.

E. The patient has *secondary* hyperparathyroidism. Surgical options should not be considered when the hyperparathyroidism can be reversed by replacement of vitamin D.

14. **C. This patient most likely has Cushing's syndrome on the basis of a functioning adrenal adenoma or carcinoma, and this should be confirmed with a CT scan of the abdomen.**

A & B. A and B might be appropriate if you suspected ectopic ACTH production secondary to lung cancer. ACTH levels would generally be very high in this setting.

D. An MRI of the pituitary would be appropriate if you suspected Cushing's disease. ACTH levels are generally normal or modestly increased. About two-thirds will have high-dose dexamethasone test suppressibility.

E. Ultrasound of the abdomen (not the pelvis) might show the adrenal glands, but a CT scan is the preferred test.

15. **A. Patients with reflux disease should be counseled on lifestyle changes that decrease the incidence of reflux, including stopping cigarette smoking and alcohol intake, reducing fat in the diet, avoiding meals 2 hours before lying down, and sleeping with the head of the bed elevated. This is the first step in managing a patient's GERD.**

B. Positive *Helicobacter pylori* serologies may indicate that a patient has a current infection, or that they have previously been infected with the organism. It is not recommended that this serology be obtained when evaluating a patient for classic GERD.

C. Promotility agents are sometimes added to a regimen of acid suppression therapy for GERD that is refractory to acid suppression therapy alone. Cisapride, the promotility agent studied most extensively in GERD, was recently restricted because of the possibility of fatal cardiac dysrhythmias due to the side effect of QT prolongation. Other promotility agents, such as metoclopramide, also have side effects, though not as severe, that may limit their use in patients.

D. Reflux of barium during radiographic evaluation is only positive in 25–75% of symptomatic patients, and is falsely positive in 20% of normal controls. Ambulatory pH testing is the best method to study the actual amount of reflux occurring in a given patient. Usually empiric acid suppression therapy is given to a patient (after lifestyle modification counseling), and the ambulatory pH testing is not needed.

E. Endoscopy should be the initial step in evaluating a patient with persistent GERD symptoms who is over 45 years of age to evaluate for premalignant lesions such as Barrett's esophagus. It should also be done in patients with alarm symptoms such as weight loss, recurrent vomiting, dysphagia, evidence of bleeding, or anemia. Our patient is 30 years old with a 3-month history of classic GERD and no alarm symptoms. Therefore, endoscopy is not initially needed.

16. **B. There is no need for any therapy or workup at this time. It takes 36–48 hours of attachment for the *Ixodes scapularis* tick to spread *Borrelia burgdorferi* to a human host. Furthermore, only 1.2–1.4% of patients bitten by *Ixodes* ticks ever develop Lyme disease. In this patient, it is unclear whether or not she was bitten at all. Therefore, she should be instructed to report any changes in her health, but further workup or therapy is not indicated in an asymptomatic patient who may or may not have been bitten by a tick.**

A. A meta-analysis of patients who were definitely bitten by an *Ixodes* tick did not show a statistically significant benefit to antibiotic prophylaxis. (Warshafsky, et al., Efficacy of antibiotic prophylaxis for prevention of Lyme disease: A meta-analysis. J Gen Intern Med 1996;11:329.) It is not even clear that this patient was bitten, so antibiotics would be inappropriate.

C. The ELISA test for *Borrelia* antibodies does not usually become positive until 6–8 weeks after exposure. A positive result immediately after a tick bite would reflect either prior exposure or false seropositivity, not evidence of current infection.

D. The indication for administration of the vaccine for Lyme disease is in individuals at high risk for exposure to the *Ixodes* tick. The United States Advisory Committee on Immunization Practices has recommended that "vaccination should be considered for patients 15–70 years of age who live, work, and recreate in high- or moderate-risk areas and are exposed to ticks either frequently or for long periods of time." (Recommendations for the use of Lyme disease vaccine. Recommendations of the Advisory Committee on Immunization Practices. MMWR Morb Mortal Wkly Rep 1999;48:1)

E. This patient is asymptomatic and stable; there is no indication for intravenous antibiotics.

17. **B. This patient has a case of traveler's diarrhea, which usually results from ingestion of contaminated food or drink while traveling to an endemic area with unsafe food and water handling. The most common organism causing this problem is enterotoxigenic *E. coli*. It results in a toxin-mediated, large volume watery diarrhea that is generally self-limited.**

A. *C. difficile* toxin can also produce a watery diarrhea with crampy abdominal pain and sometimes fever. But it is most often associated with prior antibiotic use or hospitalization.

C. *Giardia* colonizes the small intestine, leading to chronic diarrhea and/or abdominal discomfort from malabsorption. This infection is most commonly seen in patients who have been camping or drinking well water.

D. *S. typhi* causes a protracted illness with fever, headache, and splenomegaly. It more often results in constipation than diarrhea.

E. Ulcerative colitis is an autoimmune disease of the colon, resulting in mucosal inflammation and ulceration. This disease may include weight loss, bloody stools, and systemic symptoms like arthritis or rashes. The abrupt onset and otherwise benign course of this patient's presentation makes UC unlikely.

18. **C. This patient has a symptomatic urinary tract infection that needs to be treated. Amoxicillin covers the majority of the likely causative organisms, which are mainly gram-negative rods from the lower GI tract, like *E. coli*. It is safe to use in pregnancy.**

A. Fluoroquinolones should be avoided during pregnancy; they are class "C" drugs. Furthermore, a UTI during pregnancy can be more serious than in a nonpregnant woman, so it should be treated for 7 days.

B. This patient is not ill enough to require IV antibiotics.

D. Therapy can be started empirically; it is not necessary to wait for culture results.

E. A patient with a symptomatic UTI should be treated with antibiotics, regardless of whether or not she has a fever. During pregnancy, all patients with a urinalysis or urine culture positive for infection should be treated, even if they are asymptomatic.

19. A. This patient has the restrictive lung pattern and decreased gas diffusion classic of interstitial lung disease. The fact that his symptoms improve when he is away from the farm suggests an occupationally related hypersensitivity pneumonitis. Farmer's lung is a hypersensitivity reaction to thermophilic actinomycetes.

    B. COPD has an obstructive pattern on pulmonary function tests.

    C. Acute coccidioidomycosis infection would not show this restrictive lung pattern. Furthermore, the patient had symptoms prior to his Arizona trip.

    D. A reactivation of latent TB would not typically show these pulmonary function test results. Also, the chest x-ray would normally show cavitary lesions in the lung apices.

    E. Although beta-blockers can occasionally cause interstitial lung disease, the patient's symptoms would not likely improve while traveling.

20. A. This patient has a classical presentation for primary pulmonary hypertension. She will need an extensive evaluation to confirm your diagnosis and to rule out secondary causes of pulmonary hypertension (such as chronic pulmonary emboli, intrinsic lung disease, and autoimmune disorders). The therapy for pulmonary hypertension usually entails careful administration of calcium channel blockers, oxygen, and warfarin. Continuous administration of IV prostaglandin (Flolan) is also beneficial in some patients.

    B. The use of beta-blockers is not indicated in primary pulmonary hypertension. Agents which lower systemic blood pressure should be used cautiously, if at all, unless they can be shown to preferentially lower pulmonary artery pressures. While calcium channel blockers have been shown to achieve this goal in some patients, beta blockers and ACE inhibitors have not. If the systemic pressures are lowered too much, the pulmonary pressures may be so high that the RV can't fill, inducing a downward spiral in pressures and death.

    C. C is incorrect by the same rationale as outlined in B.

    D. The patient is appropriately somewhat anxious about her symptoms, but anxiety and depression do not fully explain her EKG, chest x-ray, and physical findings. While she may benefit from medications that help her cope with the poor prognosis of this disorder, answer A is clearly the single best selection for patients with primary pulmonary hypertension. PPH symptoms are often misinterpreted in young female patients for months before the true diagnosis is entertained.

    E. These would be appropriate for allergic rhinitis, not primary pulmonary hypertension.